# 基础护理技能操作指导
# （中英双语版）

# A Manual of Fundamental Nursing Skills
# （Chinese-English Edition）

主　编　练正梅

ZHEJIANG UNIVERSITY PRESS
浙江大学出版社

# A Manual of Fundamental Nursing Skills
## （Chinese-English Edition）

# 基础护理技能操作指导
## （中英双语版）
### 编委会名单

主　　编　练正梅

副 主 编　楼　艳　王　钰　张沛情

编　　委　陈婧婧　富　静　练正花

　　　　　吴小山　Agnieszka Dudek

　　　　　Theresa Abriol Santos Briones

插　　图　练正梅　魏佳禾　吴韦江

示　　教　楼　艳　陶　军　叶铭惠

演　　播　戴碧莲　高佳丽　韩妙荣　胡学高

　　　　　季绍珍　楼　艳　陶　军　吴小山

　　　　　杨梦琴　尹厚宁　游俊馨　张　婷

　　　　　周丁怡　朱凌瑜

视频拍摄　华国盛　陶　军　吴韦江

配　　音　练正梅（英文配音）　王　钰（中文配音）

字　　幕　练正梅　吴韦江

剪　　辑　吴韦江

# 序

　　中外合作办学是我国高等教育国际化发展的重要形式。为满足全球化的需要,各护理院校陆续开展中外合作办学,以培养具有国际意识、具备国际交往和国际竞争能力的高素质护理人才。丽水学院医学与健康学院积极推动护理教育国际化,于2014年与瑞典耶夫勒大学医学院合作举办护理学专业本科教育项目。在该项目实施过程中,基于双语教学的需要,基础护理学教师编写了此教材。

　　此教材英语表达专业、规范,中文表达精练,便于读者准确理解英文内容;护理程序贯穿护理技能操作全过程,符合整体护理的工作理念和方法;清晰、详细地阐述各项技能操作流程并说明其依据,为读者解难释疑;每项操作之后附注英语生词,部分生词配有构词法,帮助读者掌握构词规律,便于记忆;中、英文两套配音的操作视频,提高了教材的直观性,扩大了教材的适用群体。另外,英文配音版本添加了双语字幕,有助于读者更好地理解和掌握其中含义。

　　此教材体现了国际护理教育理念和双语教学的特点,既可用于护理学专业双语(全英文)教学,又可作为护理学专业学生英语能力训练的辅助教材,适合护理学专业学生、留学生、在职医护人员和有志于从事国际护理工作的护理人员阅读。这是一本系统、全面的优秀双语教材,特向广大护理工作者和护理学专业学生推荐。

教育部高等学校护理专业教学指导委员会秘书长

北京大学护理学院

**孙宏玉**

# 前　言

　　基础护理学实践涉及病人的健康、安全、舒适、自尊、隐私,病人与医务人员之间的沟通与合作等,在整个护理职业教育中占据重要地位。随着护理教育国际化,护理人才交流国际化,护士岗位国际化,我国各护理院校陆续开设了中外合作护理学专业。为满足护理学专业双语(全英文)教学的需求,我们在尊重英语国家语言习惯的基础上,结合我国护理操作流程,编写了《基础护理技能操作指导(中英双语版)》。

　　本教材旨在培养学生基础护理操作能力的同时,融入国外先进的护理教育理念,充分尊重病人自尊和隐私,体现人文关怀,强调节力原理在护理工作中的应用,以保护病人和医护工作者的安全;引导学生从单纯地获得技能转向提供人性化的以人为中心的服务,培养既能适应国内医疗机构的工作环境,又能适应外资医院或国外医疗机构的工作环境,具有较强国际竞争力的高素质护理人才。

　　配套视频旨在更好地帮助学生进行"基础护理学"课程的学习。

　　在此教材出版之际,我要感谢丽水学院医学与健康学院的支持,感谢丽水市第二人民医院对于视频拍摄的大力协助,感谢为此教材的出版付出辛勤努力的全体成员(尤其是叶铭惠、陶军和吴韦江),最后感谢家人给予我的理解和支持。

　　由于编者水平及各方面条件的限制,书中难免有不当及疏漏之处,敬请护理同仁及同学们不吝指正,使这本教材不断完善。

练正梅

2019 年 6 月 25 日

# CONTENTS
# 目 录

**SKILL 1   Performing Hand Hygiene**
技能操作 1　七步洗手法 ……………………………………………………………… 1

**SKILL 2   Establishing and Maintaining a Sterile Field**
技能操作 2　铺无菌盘法 ……………………………………………………………… 7

**SKILL 3   Donning and Removing Sterile Gloves**
技能操作 3　戴脱无菌手套法 ……………………………………………………… 16

**SKILL 4   Donning and Removing an Isolation Gown**
技能操作 4　穿脱隔离衣法 ………………………………………………………… 23

**SKILL 5   Making Beds**
技能操作 5　铺床法 ………………………………………………………………… 30

　　5-1　Making an Unoccupied Closed Bed
　　　　铺备用床法 ………………………………………………………………… 31

　　5-2　Making an Unoccupied Open Bed
　　　　铺暂空床法 ………………………………………………………………… 36

　　5-3　Making a Surgical Bed
　　　　铺麻醉床法 ………………………………………………………………… 36

**SKILL 6   Changing an Occupied Bed**
技能操作 6　卧床病人更换床单法 ………………………………………………… 40

**SKILL 7   Moving a Patient Up in Bed**
技能操作 7　协助病人移向床头法 ………………………………………………… 46

**SKILL 8   Turning a Patient to a Lateral Position in Bed**
技能操作 8　协助病人翻身侧卧法 ………………………………………………… 51

**SKILL 9   Mouth Care**
技能操作 9　口腔护理 ……………………………………………………………… 55

**SKILL 10   Assessing Vital Signs**
技能操作 10　生命体征测量法 ……………………………………………………… 59

　　10-1　Assessing Body Temperature
　　　　　体温测量法 ……………………………………………………………… 59

10-2　Assessing Peripheral Pulse
脉搏测量法 ·········································································· 63

10-3　Assessing Respiration
呼吸测量法 ·········································································· 66

10-4　Assessing Blood Pressure
血压测量法 ·········································································· 68

**SKILL 11　Suctioning Secretions after Tracheostomy**
技能操作 11　气管切开套管内吸痰法 ········································ 75

**SKILL 12　Administering Oxygen by Cannula or Face Mask**
技能操作 12　鼻导管、面罩吸氧法 ·········································· 82

**SKILL 13　Inserting a Nasogastric Tube and Administering Tube Feeding**
技能操作 13　插鼻胃管及鼻饲法 ············································· 89

**SKILL 14　Indwelling Urinary Catheterization**
技能操作 14　留置导尿术 ······················································· 98

**SKILL 15　Withdrawing Medication from Ampules**
技能操作 15　自安瓿抽吸药液法 ············································· 106

**SKILL 16　Withdrawing Medication from Vials**
技能操作 16　自密封瓶抽吸药液法 ········································· 110

**SKILL 17　Administering an Intradermal Injection for Skin Tests**
技能操作 17　皮内注射药物过敏试验法 ··································· 114

**SKILL 18　Administering an Intramuscular Injection**
技能操作 18　肌内注射法 ······················································· 118

**SKILL 19　Administering an Intravenous Injection**
技能操作 19　静脉注射法 ······················································· 123

**SKILL 20　Administering Peripheral Intravenous Infusion**
技能操作 20　外周静脉输液法 ················································ 129

**References**
参考文献 ·············································································· 137

# SKILL 1
# Performing Hand Hygiene

# 技能操作 1
# 七步洗手法

Health care-associated infection（HCAI）is the most common adverse event that affects hospitalized patients. Health-care workers'（HCWs）hands are considered the most important vehicle of transmitting pathogenic microorganisms to a host. WHO guidelines on patient safety（2009）addressed that sufficient hand hygiene is the most effective measure to reduce HCAI. Hand hygiene is mandatory and is a central skill for all HCWs. This is a technique of competency, professionalism and respect. Hand hygiene must be mastered by every HCW and be performed conscientiously to ensure patients' and HCWs' safety.

医源性感染是影响住院病人的最常见的不良事件。医务人员的手是传播致病微生物的最重要的媒介。2009 年，WHO 关于病人安全的指南中提出，洗手是预防医源性感染的最有效的措施。洗手法是一项核心的、必需的操作技术，是一项有关能力、专业和尊重的操作技术。医务人员必须掌握这项技术，认真洗手以确保病人和医务人员自身的安全。

二维码 1-1

二维码 1-2

## PURPOSES

1. To remove dirt and reduce microorganisms on the hands.

2. To prevent transmission of infectious organisms from nurses' hands to patients.

## ASSESSMENT

1. Determine the indications for hand hygiene. Indications for hand hygiene have been defined by the WHO（2009）：

（1）Before and after touching the patient.

（2）Moving from a contaminated body site to a clean body site during the care of the same patient.

（3）Before and after touching mucous membranes, non-intact skin, or wounds.

## 目的

1. 清除手部皮肤污垢，减少微生物数量。

2. 防止传染性微生物通过护士的手传播给病人。

## 评估

1. 确定洗手指征。2009 年 WHO 定义的洗手指征如下：

（1）直接接触病人前后。

（2）从同一病人身体的污染部位移至清洁部位时。

（3）接触病人黏膜、破损皮肤或伤口前后。

（4）After touching blood, other body fluids, secretions, excretions or wound dressings.

（5）After touching objects in the immediate vicinity of the patient(including medical equipment).

（6）Before and after putting on or removing an isolation gown.

（7）After removing sterile or non-sterile gloves.

（8）Before performing an aseptic procedure.

（9）Before handling medication or preparing food.

2. Determine hand hygiene technique:

（1）Handwashing with soap and running water must be used when the hands are:

① Visibly dirty or visibly contaminated with blood or other body fluids;

② Visibly contaminated with proteinaceous materials;

③ After touching spore-forming organisms;

④ After going to the toilet.

（2）Alcohol-based hand rub is preferred for routine hand antisepsis and when there is no visible contamination.

Advantages of alcohol-based hand rub:

① It kills bacteria more quickly and effectively;

② It causes less damage and irritation to skin;

③ It takes less time;

④ Its bottles can be placed as required so that they are more accessible.

## PLANNING

### Equipment

    1. Running water

    2. Soap or its substitutes (e. g. , liquid soap)

    3. Paper towels

    4. Alcohol-based hand rub

## IMPLEMENTATION

### Preparation

    1. Trim fingernails. **Rationale**: *Short nails are less likely to harbor microorganisms, scratch patients, or puncture gloves.*

（4）接触病人血液、其他体液、分泌物、排泄物、伤口敷料后。

（5）接触病人周围物品(包括医疗器械)后。

（6）穿脱隔离衣前后。

（7）脱手套后。

（8）无菌操作前。

（9）处理药物或配餐前。

2.确定洗手方法:

（1）以下情形须用肥皂和流动水洗手:

①有可见脏污或可见的血液、其他体液污染时;

②有可见的蛋白性物质污染时;

③接触含芽孢的物品后;

④使用洗手间后。

（2）常规手消毒或无可见污染物时首选速干手消毒剂洗手。

速干手消毒剂洗手的优点:

①能快速有效杀灭细菌;

②对皮肤的伤害和刺激性小;

③洗手快,节省时间;

④消毒剂瓶子可按需放置,方便取用。

## 计划

### 用物准备

    1.流动水

    2.肥皂或代用品(如洗手液)

    3.擦手纸

    4.速干手消毒剂

## 实施

### 准备

    1.修剪指甲。**依据**:短指甲不易藏匿病原微生物、抓伤病人或戳破手套。

2. Check hands for skin damage. **Rationale**：*A nurse who has open sores may increase the chance of acquiring or passing on an infection.*

3. Remove all jewelry. **Rationale**：*Microorganisms can paratise jewelry, such as rings. Removal facilitates proper cleaning of the hands and arms.*

4. Roll the sleeves up if needed.

## Procedure

### Handwashing with running water

1. Turn on the faucet and adjust it to warm water. **Rationale**：*Warm water is less likely to remove the protective oil of the skin than hot water.*

2. Wet the hands thoroughly under the running water from the lower forearms to the fingertips. **Rationale**：*The water should flow from the least contaminated area to the most contaminated area; the hands are generally considered more contaminated than the lower forearms.*

3. Apply 4-5 mL liquid soap to hands. If it is a bar soap, rub it firmly between the hands.

Use firm and circular rubbing movements to wash the palm, back, and wrist of each hand. Be sure to include the heel of the hands. Interlace the fingers, and move the hands back and forth. The WHO (2009) recommends these steps (see Figure 1-1 (a)-(g))：

(1) Rub hands palm to palm.

(2) Right palm over left dorsum with interlaced fingers and vice versa.

(3) Palm to palm with fingers interlaced.

(4) Backs of fingers to opposing palms with fingers interlocked.

(5) Rotational rubbing of left thumb clasped in right palm and vice versa.

(6) Rotational rubbing, backwards and forwards

2. 检查双手有无破损。**依据**：若护士双手有开放性损伤，可增加获得感染或传播感染的概率。

3. 取下手上饰物。**依据**：微生物可寄生于首饰中，如戒指；取下饰物，方便洗手。

4. 必要时拉高衣袖。

## 操作步骤

### 流动水洗手法

1. 打开水龙头，调至温水。**依据**：温水较热水不易洗去皮肤上的保护性油脂。

2. 在流动水下，从前臂向下，充分淋湿双手。**依据**：水应从轻度污染区流向重度污染区，一般情况下，双手比前臂污染严重。

3. 取 4~5 mL 洗手液。如为肥皂块，应用力揉搓肥皂。

以旋转式动作用力揉搓手掌、手背、手腕、掌跟，交叉手指，来回揉搓。2009 年 WHO 建议的洗手步骤如下（见图 1-1 (a)~(g)）：

(1) 手指并拢，掌心相对，相互揉搓。

(2) 掌心对手背沿指缝揉搓，交换进行。

(3) 掌心相对，双手交叉沿指缝相互揉搓。

(4) 弯曲手指使关节在另一掌心旋转揉搓，交换进行。

(5) 右手握住左手大拇指，回旋揉搓，交换进行。

(6) 五个手指尖并拢在另一

with clasped fingertips of right hand in left palm and vice versa. **Rationale**：*The nails and fingertips are usually missed during hand hygiene.*

掌心旋转揉搓,交换进行。**依据**：洗手时指甲和指尖部分常被忽略。

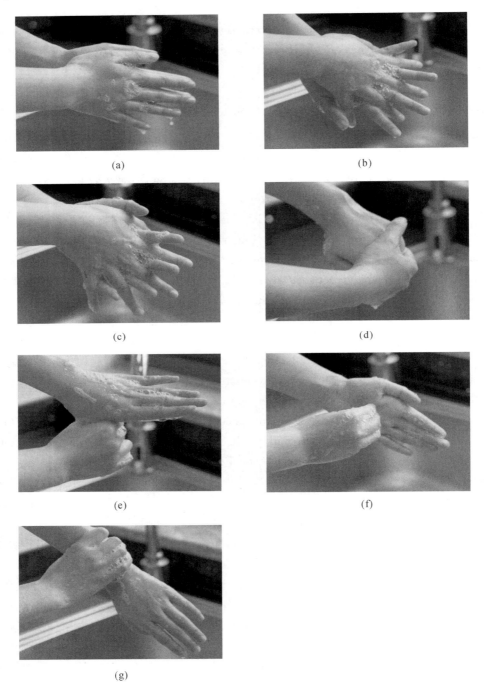

(a)　　　　　　　　　　　(b)

(c)　　　　　　　　　　　(d)

(e)　　　　　　　　　　　(f)

(g)

Figure 1-1　Handwashing steps

图 1-1　洗手步骤

（7）Rotational rubbing of left wrist claspled in right palm and vice versa. Continue these motions for about 30 seconds.

4. Rinse hands with running water thoroughly.

5. Dry hands and arms with a single-use paper towel. Gently pad the skin rather than rubbing it.

6. Use a new paper towel to grasp the faucet handle to turn off the water (see Figure 1-2). **Rationale**: *This prevents the nurse from picking up microorganisms from the faucet handle.*

The entire procedure should take 40 to 60 seconds.

### Hand rubbing with alcohol-based hand rub

1. Apply about 3 mL of the product to a cupped hand and cover all surfaces of the hands.

2. Complete the hand rubbing procedure by following the procedures previously described for the handwashing procedure with running water until the hands become dry. This rubbing procedure takes about 20 to 30 seconds.

## EVALUATION

• There is no conventional evaluation of the effectiveness of handwashing practice. More attention should be paid on HCWs adherence to the recommended hand hygiene procedures.

（7）右手握住左手手腕，回旋揉搓，交换进行，揉搓约 30 秒。

4. 在流动水下彻底冲净双手。

5. 用一次性擦手纸擦干双手，勿用力擦。

6. 如水龙头为手开式开关，应用干净纸巾垫着把手关闭水龙头（见图 1-2）。**依据**：避免双手再次被污染。

整个洗手过程需 40～60 秒。

### 速干手消毒剂洗手法

1. 取速干手消毒剂约 3 mL，涂满双手。

2. 同流动水洗手法搓手至消毒剂干燥。整个搓手过程需 20～30 秒。

## 评价

• 对洗手效果没有常规评价方法，应重点关注医务人员是否按规定程序进行有效洗手。

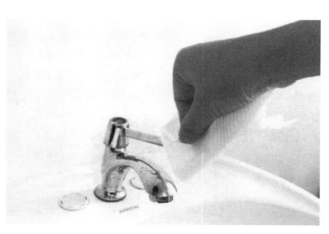

Figure 1-2　Using a paper towel to grasp the handle of a hand-operated faucet

图 1-2　用纸巾垫着打开手开式水龙头

# Words and Expressions

accessible *adj.* 可接近的,可使用的

adherence *n.* 遵循,遵守

adverse *adj.* 相反的,不利的

alcohol *n.* 酒精,乙醇

antisepsis *n.* 抗菌,防腐

aseptic *adj.* 无(病)菌的

　　(前缀 a-, an- 表示"无,不")

aseptic technique 无菌技术

bacteria *n.* 细菌

bend *v.* (使四肢等)弯曲,把……弄弯,折起

circular *adj.* 圆形的,环形的

contaminate *vt.* 污染,弄脏

contamination *n.* 污染

conventional *adj.* 传统的,习惯的

determine *vt.* 决定,确定,判定

dorsum *n.* 背部,背侧

ensure *vt.* 保证,确保

excrete *vt.* 排泄

excretion *n.* 排泄,排泄物

facilitate *vt.* 促进,促使,使便利

faucet *n.* 水龙头

forearm *n.* 前臂

handle *n.* 把手,拉手;*vt.* 处理,控制

harbor *vi.* 藏有,包含

implement *vt.* 实施,执行

implementation *n.* 实施,执行

indication *n.* 标示,象征,表明

infection *n.* 感染,传染

infectious *adj.* 感染的,传染性的

irritation *n.* 刺激,激怒,恼怒

mandatory *adj.* 强制的

membrane *n.* 膜,薄膜

microorganism *n.* 微生物

　　(前缀 micro- 表示"微,小")

organism *n.* 微生物,生物体

palm *n.* 手掌,手心

paratise *vt.* 寄宿于

pathogenic *adj.* 致病的,发病的

proteinaceous *adj.* 蛋白质的

puncture *vt.* 戳破,刺破;*vi.* 被刺破;

　　*n.* 扎孔,刺伤

rationale *n.* 理论依据;根本原因

rinse *vt.* (用清水)冲掉,洗刷

rotational *adj.* 转动的,旋转的

secrete *vt.* 分泌

secretion *n.* 分泌,分泌物

substitute *n.* 代用品,代替者

sufficient *adj.* 充足的,足够的

thoroughly *adv.* 彻底地,完全地

transmission *n.* 传播,传染

transmit *vt.* 传染,传播

　　(前缀 trans- 表示"横穿,通过")

trim *vt.* 修剪,整理

vehicle *n.* 手段,工具

vice versa 反之亦然

vicinity *n.* 邻近,附近

vigorously *adv.* 用力地,活泼地

visible *adj.* 看得见的,明显的

visibly *adv.* 明显地,易察觉地

wrist *n.* 手腕,腕关节

# SKILL 2　Establishing and Maintaining a Sterile Field

# 技能操作 2 铺无菌盘法

A sterile field is a microorganism-free area. Nurses often establish one by using the innermost side of a sterile wrapper, or a sterile drape. When the field is established, sterile supplies can be placed on it. In order to reduce the patient's risk of acquiring hospital infection, nurses must possess great awareness of aseptic environment and rigorously adhere to the principles of aseptic technique when establishing a sterile field.

无菌区是指没有病原微生物的区域。护士通常使用无菌包布的内面或无菌治疗巾来建立无菌区域。无菌区内可放置无菌物品。护士在建立无菌区时应具备很强的无菌意识，严格遵守无菌技术操作原则，以减小病人获得医院感染的概率。

二维码 2-1

二维码 2-2

## PURPOSE

• To ensure that sterile items remain sterile.

## ASSESSMENT

• Review the patient's record to determine which procedure will need a sterile field.

## PLANNING

### Equipment

1. Clean tray
2. Package containing sterile drapes
3. Sterile containers (e. g. , sterile medical stainless steel container)
4. Sterile supplies as needed (e. g. , sterile bowl, sterile gauze, sterile solution)
5. Forceps containers (wide mouth, with a cover)

## 目的

• 保持无菌物品的无菌。

## 评估

• 查看病历,确定无菌盘的用途。

## 计划

### 用物准备

1.治疗盘
2.无菌治疗巾包
3.无菌容器(如无菌贮槽)

4.所需的无菌物品(如无菌碗、无菌纱布、无菌溶液)
5.持物钳容器(带盖大口)

6. Sterile tissue forceps

7. Sterile three-toothed pick-up forceps

8. Clean bowl

9. Clean towels

## IMPLEMENTATION

### Preparation

1. Ensure that the working area is clean.

2. Perform hand hygiene, and put on a mask.

3. Ensure that the wrapped package is clean and dry. If there are stains or spots on the outside of the package or if moisture is felt, it is considered contaminated and must be disposed.

4. Check the sterilization chemical indicators and dates on the packages and containers, and look for any indications that they have been previously opened (if so, ensure their validity).

5. Wipe the outside of the unwrapped bottle with a damp towel to remove any dust that could fall into the bowl or the field.

6. Wipe the tray and working table with a clean towel.

### Procedure

1. Perform hand hygiene.

2. Open a wrapped package:

(1) Put the package on the working table so that the top flap of the wrapper is in a distal position (see Figure 2-1(a)).

(2) Reach around the package (not over it), use your thumb and index finger to pinch the first flap on the outside of the wrapper and open away from you, then open two side flaps (see Figure 2-1(b)). **Rationale**: *Touching only the outside of the wrapper maintains the sterility of the inside of the wrapper.*

3. Open the last flap with the non-dominant hand. Ensure the sterility of the drape by checking the sterilization chemical indicator.

4. With the dominant hand, use sterile three-toothed pick-up forceps to take one drape out and put

6. 无菌持物镊

7. 无菌三叉钳

8. 清洁碗

9. 清洁毛巾

## 实施

### 准备

1. 确认操作环境清洁。

2. 洗手，戴口罩。

3. 确定无菌治疗巾包布清洁干燥，包外如有污迹或包布潮湿应视为污染，不可使用。

4. 检查无菌包及无菌容器的灭菌指示卡和灭菌日期，是否曾经打开（如曾打开，应在有效期内）。

5. 用微湿毛巾擦净无包装的溶液瓶身，防止瓶外灰尘掉入无菌碗或无菌区内。

6. 用清洁毛巾擦净治疗盘和操作台面。

### 操作步骤

1. 七步洗手法洗手。

2. 打开无菌治疗巾包：

（1）将无菌治疗巾包放于操作台面上，外角在对侧（见图 2-1(a)）。

（2）用拇指和食指捏住外角的外面向对侧打开（勿跨越），然后打开左右两角（见图 2-1(b)）。**依据**：捏住外面保持包布内面无菌。

3. 用非惯用手打开最后一角。查看灭菌指示卡，确认治疗巾灭菌有效。

4. 惯用手持三叉钳夹取一块无菌治疗巾置于治疗盘内（见图

it on the treatment tray (see Figure 2-2).

5. Repack the package (if it contains more than one drape) and record the date and time of opening. It is permitted for the repacked package to be reused within 24 hours (see Figure 2-3).

2-2)。

5. 如治疗巾未用完，按要求回包，注明开包日期和时间，24小时内有效（见图 2-3）。

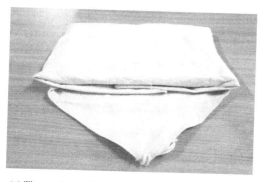

(a) The top flap of the wrapper opening away from you

(a) 包布外角在对侧

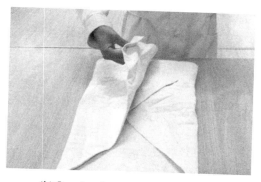

(b) Opening the second flap to the side

(b) 打开第二角

Figure 2-1　Opening the package

图 2-1　打开无菌治疗巾包

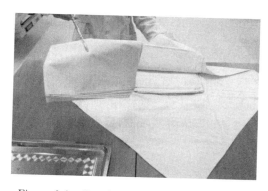

Figure 2-2　Opening the last flap by pinching and pulling it with the tip towards you

图 2-2　捏住最后一角尖外层向自己方向打开

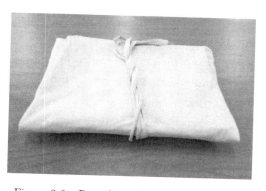

Figure 2-3　Repacking the package(if it contains more than one drape)

图 2-3　治疗巾未用完，系带一字形回包

6. Establish a sterile field by using a drape (a single layer method):

(1) Hold the outer corners of the drape (that was folded in two) and place it evenly on the tray, placing the open side distant from you (see Figure 2-4). **Rationale**: *By placing the lowermost side farthest away, you can avoid leaning over the sterile*

6. 单层底铺无菌盘法：

（1）双手捏住呈双折的治疗巾外面两角，抖开，对称地平铺于治疗盘上，开口边铺向对侧（见图 2-4）。**依据**：开口边铺向对侧可避免打开上层治疗巾时手臂跨越

field and contaminating it.

(2) Touching only the outside of the drape, hold the two far corners of the top layer with the thumb and the index finger. Fanfold it horizontally towards you, the edge of the top flap facing outwards (see Figure 2-5).

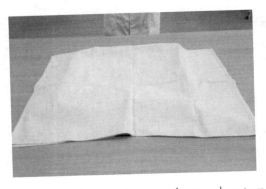

Figure 2-4　Placing a drape evenly on a clean tray

图 2-4　治疗巾对称地平铺于治疗盘上

(3) Open the cover of the medical stainless steel container completely before taking the sterile bowl out. **Rationale**：*This reduces the likelihood of the bowl touching the rim of the cover.*

7. Add solution to a sterile bowl：

(1) Before pouring any liquid, read the label to make sure you have the right solution and concentration.

(2) Check if the lid is securely screwed.

(3) Invert the bottle to check the quality of the solution.

(4) If the bottle has not been previously opened, remove its lid, then remove the rubber stopper and hold it in your fingers (or invert the stopper before placing it on an unsterile surface). Avoid touching the rim of the bottle or the inside of the stopper with your fingers.

(5) Hold the bottle with the label facing your palm. Pour a little bit of the solution to wash the rim of the bottle. **Rationale**：*Any solution that flows down the outside of the bottle during pouring will damage the label.*

(6) Lift it at a height of 10 to 15 cm over the

无菌区。

(2)以拇指和食指捏住治疗巾上层两角的外面,扇形折向自己,开口边向外(见图 2-5)。

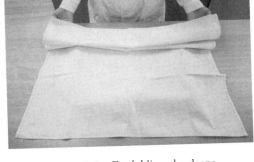

Figure 2-5　Fanfolding the drape

图 2-5　扇形折叠治疗巾

(3)夹取无菌碗前将贮槽完全打开。**依据**:减少无菌碗触及槽盖边缘的概率。

7. 倒取无菌溶液:

(1)倒溶液前先检查标签,确认溶液名称、浓度正确。

(2)检查瓶盖应拧紧。

(3)倒转瓶子检查溶液质量。

(4)如瓶子未曾打开,撬开瓶盖。打开瓶塞,拿在手指间或倒转瓶塞放于操作台面上。手指不可触及瓶口及瓶塞内面。

(5)手持溶液瓶,标签朝向掌心,倒出少许溶液旋转冲洗瓶口。**依据**:标签朝向掌心可避免溶液流至瓶身污染或损坏标签。

(6)溶液瓶在 10～15 cm 高

bowl and to the side of the field. **Rationale**：*At this height, there is less likelihood of contaminating the sterile field by touching the field or by scretching an arm over it*. Pour the solution carefully to avoid splashing the liquid （see Figure 2-6）. **Rationale**：*Moisture will contaminate the field by wicking microorganisms through the drape*.

（7） After pouring liquid, turn the bottle quickly upright to avoid the liquid flowing down the outside of the bottle. **Rationale**：*Such drips would contaminate the sterile field if the outside of the bottle is not sterile*.

（8） If the solution will be used again, replace the rubber stopper securely and document the date and time of opening and sign your full name on the label of the bottle. **Rationale**：*Replacing the lid immediately maintains the sterility of the inner side of the lid and the solution*. It is permitted for the rest solution to be reused within 24 hours.

8. Put necessary sterile supplies in the field as needed.

9. After adding all necessary sterile supplies, hold the outer corners of the upper layer to cover the sterile area （see Figure 2-7）. Then fold the opened edge twice upwards （see Figure 2-8）. Fold the side edges downwards or upwards once （see Figure 2-9）.

处对准无菌碗,从无菌区侧边,小心倒入所需液量。**依据**:此高度可防止溶液瓶触及无菌区,从无菌区侧边倒取溶液可减少跨越无菌区范围。勿使溶液溅出(见图2-6)。**依据**:潮湿的治疗巾产生毛细作用,使微生物渗入而污染无菌区。

（7）倒完溶液后迅速将瓶子竖起,防止溶液流至瓶身。**依据**:防止溶液滴落污染无菌区。

（8）如剩余溶液仍需利用,塞好瓶塞,在瓶签上注明开瓶日期、时间并签名。**依据**:倒完溶液后立即塞好瓶塞可保持剩余溶液无菌及减少瓶塞暴露时间。剩余溶液24小时内有效。

8. 在无菌区内放入所需无菌物品。

9. 放入所需无菌物品后,捏住治疗巾上层两角的外面拉平扇形折叠层,对齐边缘,遮盖物品(见图2-7)。将开口边向上反折两次(见图2-8),左右两边向下或向上反折一次,铺好无菌盘(见图2-9)。

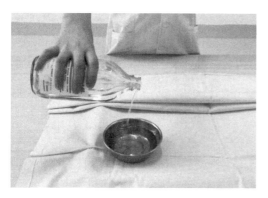

Figure 2-6   Adding a liquid to a sterile bowl
图 2-6   倒无菌溶液于无菌碗中

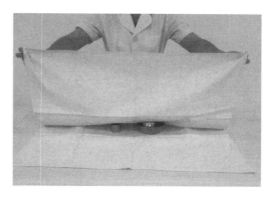

Figure 2-7   Holding the two outer corners of the upper layer to cover the sterile supplies
图 2-7   双手捏住上层治疗巾外面两角,遮盖于无菌物品上

10. Document the date and time to establish the sterile area. Sign your full name. It is permitted the sterile supplies to be used within 4 hours.

10. 记录铺盘日期、时间,签全名。盘内物品 4 小时内有效。

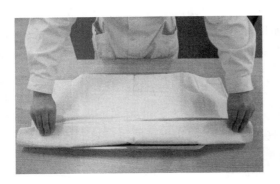

Figure 2-8　Folding upwards the opened edge twice

图 2-8　开口处向上翻折两次

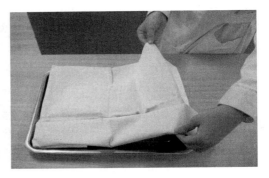

Figure 2-9　Folding downwards or upwards the side edges once

图 2-9　两侧边缘分别向下或向上翻折一次

Note：Use of sterile forceps

1. Forceps are usually used to move a sterile object from one place to another, for example, to transfer a sterile gauze from its package to a sterile dressing tray. Forceps may be disposed or sterilized again after use. Commonly used forceps include hemostats (see Figure 2-10) and tissue forceps (see Figure 2-11).

注：无菌持物钳使用法

1. 无菌持物钳用于传递无菌物品,如从无菌包中夹取无菌纱布放于无菌换药盘中。无菌持物钳有一次性及非一次性,常用的有血管钳(见图 2-10)和镊子(见图 2-11)。

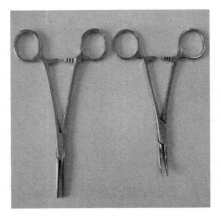

Figure 2-10　Hemostats：*Left*—straight；*Right*—curved

图 2-10　血管钳:左—直,右—弯

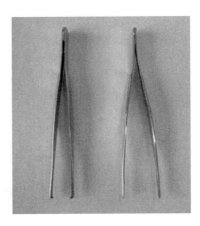

Figure 2-11　Tissue forceps：*Left*—toothed；*Right*—plain

图 2-11　镊子:左—有齿镊,右—无齿镊

2. Before taking them out, open the cover of the container, hold the upper part (at about 1/3 length from the top) and move them to the center of the container. Close the tips together and take the forceps out of the container vertically (see Figure 2-12(a),(b)). Aavoid touching the inner wall above the solution level and the rim of the container. **Rationale:** *The inner wall above the solution level is considered not absolutely sterile while the rim of the container is unsterile.*

2. 使用前先打开无菌持物钳容器盖,手持无菌持物钳上 1/3 处,将钳移至容器中央,闭合钳端,竖直取出(见图 2-12(a),(b))。钳端不可触及液面以上内壁及容器口缘。**依据**:液面以上内壁为非绝对无菌区,而容器口缘为有菌区。

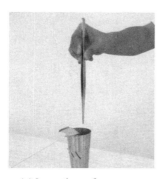 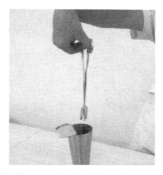

(a) Long tissue forceps　　　　　　(b) Three-toothed pick-up forceps
(a) 长镊子　　　　　　　　　　　(b) 三叉钳

Figure 2-12　Taking the sterile forceps out of the sterile container

图 2-12　从无菌持物钳容器中取出无菌持物钳

3. If the forceps are soaked in antiseptic solution, keep them in a downward position at all times, below the wrist. **Rationale:** *It prevents liquids on the tips of the forceps from flowing to the unsterile handles and later back to the tips.* Hold sterile forceps within your sight and above the waist or table surface. **Rationale:** *Items held below waist or table surface or out of sight should be considered contaminated.*

3. 若持物钳浸泡在消毒液中,使用时始终保持钳端向下、低于手腕水平。**依据**:防止钳端溶液流向未消毒的手柄,再流回钳端使其污染。持物钳应保持在视线范围内、腰部或操作台面以上。**依据**:在腰部或操作台面以下或离开视线的持物钳应视为污染。

4. After using, put the forceps back to the container vertically with tips closed and down. Loosen the joint pivot of the forceps if they are soaked in antiseptic solution (e. g., three-toothed pick-up forceps, hemostats). **Rationale:** *Loosening the joint pivot allows all surfaces of the forceps to be soaked in antiseptic solution.* Close the cover of the forceps container.

4. 用后闭合钳端,竖直放入容器中。如浸泡在消毒液中,应打开轴节(如三叉钳、血管钳)。**依据**:打开轴节使持物钳得到充分浸泡。关闭容器盖。

5. Bring the forceps together with the container when fetching sterile objects placed elsewhere. **Rationale**：*This prevents the forceps from exposing in the air too long.*

6. Put a sterile item in the sterile field without permitting wet forceps to touch the field.

## EVALUATION

● Ensure that an adequate number of and a variety of sterile supplies are available for the next HCW.

5.到远处取物时,连同容器一起搬移。**依据**:防止持物钳在空气中暴露过久。

6.在消毒液中浸泡的持物钳不可触及无菌区域。

## 评价

● 确保下一位操作者有充足的无菌物品。

# Words and Expressions

antiseptic *adj.* 防腐的,抗菌的,消毒过的
　　(前缀 anti- 表示"反对,反")
awareness *n.* 意识,认识,知道
clean/treatment tray 治疗盘
concentration *n.* 浓度;集中,关注
curved *adj.* 呈弯曲状的,弧形的
dispose *vt.* 处理,解决
distal *adj.* 远端的,末梢的
document *vt.* 记录;*n.* 文件,公文
dominant *adj.* 占支配地位的,占优势的
drape *n.* 帘子,帷幕;*vt.* 悬挂,披
evenly *adv.* 均匀地,相等地
fanfold *vt.* 扇形折叠
flap *n.* (附于某物的)片状下垂物,封盖,口盖
fold *vt.* 折叠
forceps *n.* (医用)镊子,钳子
gauze *n.* 纱布
hemostats *n.* (医用)止血钳
　　(前缀 hemo-/haemo- 表示"(有关)血液的")
horizontally *adv.* 水平地,与地平面平行地
index finger/forefinger 食指,示指
indicator *n.* 指示器,标志,迹象
inner *adj.* 内部的,内心的
innermost *adj.* 最靠近中心的,内心深处的

invert *vt.* 倒置,(使)倒转
lid *n.* (容器的)盖子
likelihood *n.* 可能性,可能
maintain *vt.* 保持,维持
moisture *n.* 潮气,水分
pinch *vt.* 捏住,夹紧
pivot *n.* 枢轴,中心点
review *vt.* 回顾,复查,复习;*n.* 回顾,审查
　　(前缀 re- 表示"重新,再,又")
rigorously *adv.* 严格地,严厉地,谨慎地
rim *n.* (圆形物体的)边沿
screw *vt.* 拧紧,旋紧
sign *vt.* 签(名),署(名),签字;*n.* 体征,迹象,征兆
splash *vt.* 把(水、泥等)溅在……上
spot *n.* 斑点,污渍,脏点
stain *n.* 污点,污渍
sterile *adj.* 无菌的,消过毒的
sterile drape 无菌治疗巾
sterile field/area 无菌区
sterile supplies/items 无菌物品
sterility *n.* 无菌
sterilization *n.* 灭菌,消毒
sterilize *vt.* 灭菌,消毒
stopper *n.* 瓶塞
tip *vi.* 尖端,末端

tissue forceps (plain, toothed) 镊子(平镊，有齿镊)

transfer *vt.* (使)转移，(使)调动

upright *adj.* 垂直的，直立的

validity *n.* (法律上的)有效，合法性

vertically *adv.* 垂直地，直立地

wick *vt.* 吸取，吸走；*n.* 灯芯，烛芯

wrap *vt.* 包，裹(礼物等)

wrapped *adj.* 有包装的

wrapper *n.* 包装纸，包装材料

# SKILL 3　Donning and Removing Sterile Gloves

Sterile gloves are worn during medical and nursing procedures to maintain the sterility of the procedure and to protect both patients and nurses.

二维码 3-1

## PURPOSES

1. To allow the nurses to handle or touch sterile items freely without contaminating them.

2. To prevent transmission of potential pathogenic organisms from the nurses' hands to patients who are at high risk of infection.

## ASSESSMENT

● Determine the purpose of wearing sterile gloves. Check the patient's record and ask about latex allergies. Use non-latex sterile gloves if necessary.

## PLANNING

● Be well planned. Make sure all preparations are completed before putting on the gloves. Prepare an extra pair of sterile gloves.

### Equipment

● Sterile gloves of the right size

## IMPLEMENTATION

### Preparation

1. Trim fingernails.

2. Remove all jewelry from the hands.

# 技能操作 3　戴脱无菌手套法

在医疗和护理操作过程中戴无菌手套以保持操作中的无菌，同时保护病人和护士。

二维码 3-2

## 目的

1. 便于护士随意触碰无菌物品而不使其污染。

2. 防止潜在的病原微生物通过护士的双手传播给易感病人。

## 评估

● 确定戴无菌手套的目的。查看病历或询问病人是否对乳胶过敏，如有过敏，应使用非乳胶手套。

## 计划

● 计划周详，操作前确定用物齐全，准备一副备用手套。

### 用物准备

● 型号合适的无菌手套

## 实施

### 准备

1. 修剪指甲。

2. 取下手上饰物。

## Procedure

**To don sterile gloves**

▶ Mothod 1

1. Perform hand hygiene, and put on a mask.

2. Ensure the sterility of the gloves (ensure that cloth-wrapped package is clean and dry).

3. Open the package of the sterile gloves:

(1) Place the package of gloves on a clean, dry surface. **Rationale**: *Any moisture on the surface could contaminate the gloves.*

(2) If the gloves are packaged with an outer and an inner layers, open the outer package without contaminating the gloves.

(3) Take out the inner package from the outer package.

(4) Open the inner package carefully. Do not touch the inner surface. **Rationale**: *The inner surface, which is next to the sterile gloves, should remain sterile.*

4. Pick up the gloves by holding the two cuffs with the thumb and the index finger of one hand. Avoid contaminating the outer side of the gloves (see Figure 3-1).

5. Put on the first glove for the dominant hand:

Insert the dominant hand into the glove and pull on the glove while the non-dominant hand is holding both cuffs. Leave the cuff in place once the non-dominant hand releases the glove (see Figure 3-2). **Rationale**: *In this position, it is less likely to contaminate the outside of the glove.*

6. Put on the second glove for the nondominant hand:

(1) Insert four fingers of the gloved hand under the cuff while holding the gloved thumb as far away from the palm as possible (see Figures 3-3, 3-4). **Rationale**: *In this position, the thumb is less likely to touch the cuff of the other glove and become contaminated.* Put on the second glove carefully.

## 操作步骤

**戴无菌手套法**

▶方法一

1. 洗手,戴口罩。

2. 确定手套的无菌性(包布应清洁干燥)。

3. 打开无菌手套包:

(1)将手套包装袋放于清洁、干燥的操作台面上。**依据**:台面潮湿将致手套污染。

(2)如是双层包装,打开外层包装时勿污染手套。

(3)从外层包装中取出内层包装。

(4)小心打开内层包装,勿触及包装层内面。**依据**:包装层内面因与无菌手套接触,所以应保持无菌。

4. 用一手拇指和食指同时捏住两只手套的反折部分,取出手套,勿污染手套外面(见图3-1)。

5. 戴惯用手手套:

非惯用手捏住两只手套的反折部分,惯用手伸入右手套内,五指对准拉上。非惯用手放开,勿将反折部分翻上(见图3-2)。**依据**:降低污染手套外面的概率。

6. 戴非惯用手手套:

(1)将已戴手套的四个手指插入另一手套反折部分的内面(手套外面),拇指尽量向外伸展,远离手掌(见图3-3、图3-4)。**依据**:戴了手套的拇指远离手掌可降低触及另一手套反折部分而被污染的概率。小心戴好非惯用手手套。

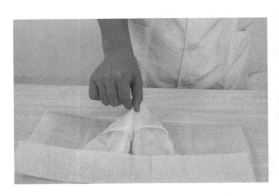

Figure 3-1　Picking up a pair of sterile gloves with one hand

图 3-1　单手取出无菌手套

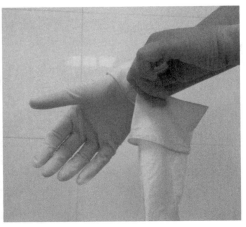

Figure 3-2　Putting on the first glove, leaving the cuff in place

图 3-2　戴上第一只手套后,勿将反折部上翻

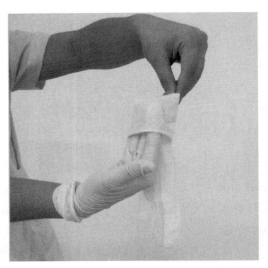

Figure 3-3　Inserting the gloved fingers under the cuff while streching the thumb of the gloved hand away from the palm

图 3-3　戴好手套的手指插入另一手套的反折内面,拇指向外伸展远离手掌

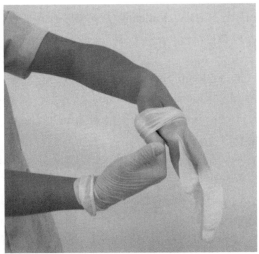

Figure 3-4　Putting on the second sterile glove

图 3-4　戴第二只手套

（2）Unfold the glove cuff of the non-dominant hand and then that of the dominant one（see Figure 3-5）.

（2）将非惯用手手套反折部翻上,再翻惯用手手套（见图 3-5）。

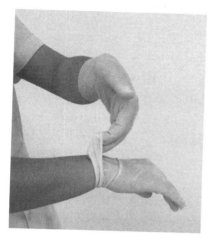

Figure 3-5　Unfolding the cuffs

图 3-5　上翻手套反折部

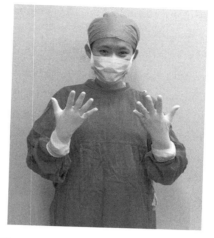

Figure 3-6　Cuffs of the gloves covering
the cuffs of the gown

图 3-6　手套的反折部上翻扣套在衣袖外面

（3）If you wear a gown, pull the gloves up to cover the cuffs of the gown（see Figure 3-6）. If you do not wear a gown, pull the cuffs of the gloves up to cover the wrists. Check the intactness of the gloves. Adjust each glove so that it fits comfortably.

▶Mothod 2

After opening the package:

1. Put on the first glove for the dominant hand:

（1）Grasp the glove for the dominant hand by its folded cuff edge（on the side of the palm）with the thumb and first finger of the non-dominant hand. Touch only the inside of the cuff（see Figure 3-7）.

（2）Insert the dominant hand into the glove and pull on the glove. Leave the cuff in place once the non-dominant hand releases the glove（see Figure 3-2）.

（3）如穿长袖工作服,手套翻边应扣套在工作服袖口外（见图3-6）,穿短袖时翻边则遮盖手腕处。检查手套有无破损,调整手套至服帖。

▶方法二

打开手套包后:

1.戴惯用手手套:

（1）用非惯用手拇指和食指捏住惯用手手套反折部（掌侧）取出手套。只能触及反折部内面（见图3-7）。

（2）惯用手对准五指戴上手套。放开非惯用手,勿将反折部分翻上（见图3-2）。

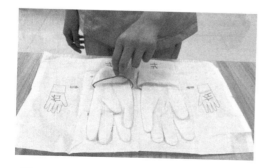

Figure 3-7　Picking up the first sterile glove

图 3-7　取第一只手套

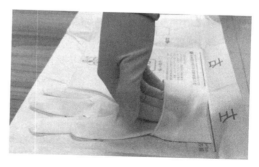

Figure 3-8　Picking up the second sterile glove

图 3-8　取第二只手套

2. Put on the second glove for the non-dominant hand：

（1）Pick up the other glove with the gloved hand, insert the gloved four fingers under the cuff (see Figure 3-8) and put on the second glove carefully (see Figures 3-3, 3-4).

（2）Unfold the glove cuffs of the nondominant hand and then the dominant one (see Figure 3-5).

**To remove the gloves**

▶Mothod 1

1. Grasp the palmar surface of the first glove, and take off the glove by turning it inside out. Make sure that the outside of the gloves do not touch your skin or uniform (see Figure 3-9).

2.戴非惯用手手套：

（1）用戴了手套的四个手指插入左手手套的反折部内面取出手套（见图 3-8），小心戴好左手手套（见图 3-3、图 3-4）。

（2）将左手手套反折部翻上，再翻右手手套（见图 3-5）。

**脱手套法**

▶方法一

1.用戴着手套的手捏住另一手套口掌侧外面，将手套翻转脱下，使手套污染面翻向内面。手套外面勿触及皮肤或工作服（见图 3-9）。

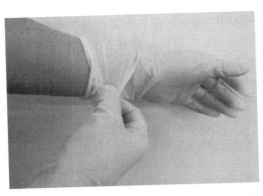

Figure 3-9　Grasping the palmar surface of the first contaminated glove

图 3-9　捏住污染的手套口掌侧外面

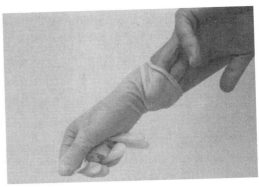

Figure 3-10　Inserting the fingers of the bare hand inside the cuff

图 3-10　脱下手套的手指插入另一手套内

2. Hold the removed glove by the gloved hand and insert fingers or the thumb of the bare hand inside the cuff (see Figures 3-10, 3-11). Then remove the second glove completely by turning it inside out and wrap the first glove in the second one (see Figures 3-12, 3-13). **Rationale**：*Wrap the soiled side of the gloves inside to reduce the chance of transferring microorganisms by direct contact.*

2.用戴着手套的手抓住已脱下的手套，将已脱手套的手指伸入另一手套内（见图 3-10、图 3-11），同法将手套内面向外翻转脱下，包住已脱下的手套（见图 3-12、图 3-13）。**依据**：手套污染面翻至内面以降低通过直接接触传播微生物的概率。

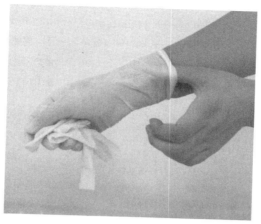

Figure 3-11　Inserting the thumb of the bare hand inside the cuff (resembling a hook)

图 3-11　脱下手套的手拇指插入另一手套内(似钩状)

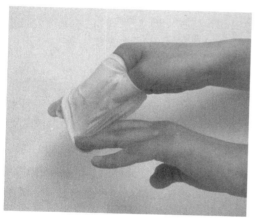

Figure 3-12　Removing the second glove by turning it inside out to keep the soiled part of the gloves inside

图 3-12　第二只手套翻转脱下后将两只手套的污染面包裹在内

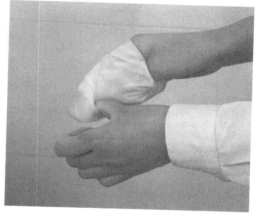

Figure 3-13　Wrapping the first glove in the second one

图 3-13　第二只手套包裹第一只手套

▶Mothod 2

1. Grasp the palmar surface of the first glove, and pull the glove down by turning it inside out until the thumb comes out. Make sure that the outside of the gloves do not touch your skin or uniform (see Figure 3-9).

2. Insert the thumb of the first hand (resemb-

▶方法二

1.用戴着手套的手捏住另一手套口掌侧外面,将手套翻转脱至拇指完全露出,手套外面勿触及皮肤或工作服(见图 3-9)。

2.将已露出手套的拇指伸入

ling a hook) inside the cuff of the second glove (see Figure 3-14). Remove the second glove completely by turning it inside out, then the first one. This makes the two gloves removed separately (see Figure 3-15).

另一手套内（似钩状）（见图 3-14）；将手套内面向外翻转脱下，再将第一只手套完全脱下。此法使两只手套分开脱下（见图 3-15）。

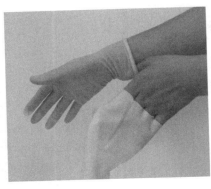

Figure 3-14　Inserting the exposed thumb inside the cuff

图 3-14　露出的手拇指插入另一手套内

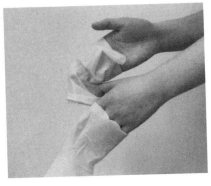

Figure 3-15　Removing the gloves separately by turning them inside out

图 3-15　两只手套分开脱下

3. Dispose the gloves appropriately.

4. Perform hand hygiene.

5. Document that the sterile technique was used during the procedure.

3.妥善弃置手套。

4.洗手。

5.记录。

## EVALUATION

• Check the gloves are intact and not contaminated during the procedure.

## 评价

• 手套完整无破损，操作过程无污染。

## Words and Expressions

allergy *n.* 过敏反应，变态反应

appropriately *adv.* 适当地，合适地

cuff *n.* 袖口，(裤脚的)外翻边，外卷边

glove *n.* 手套

grasp *vt.* 抓紧，抓牢，领会，理解

insert *vt.* 插入

intact *adj.* 完整的，完好无损的

latex *n.* (天然)乳胶

potential *adj.* 可能的，潜在的

resemble *vt.* 像，看起来像，显得像

soil *vt.* 弄脏；*n.* 土壤，领土，土地

unfold *vt.* 打开，(使)展开

　　(前缀 un- 表示"不，未，非，反")

wear *v.* 穿，戴(过去分词 worn)

# SKILL 4   Donning and Removing an Isolation Gown

When caring for isolated patients, in order to protect patients and HCWs and to avoid cross-infection, nurses need to wear isolation gowns.

二维码 4-1

## PURPOSE

- To protect HCWs and patients from transmission of potentially infectious materials (e. g., blood, other body fluids).

## ASSESSMENT

- Assess the patient's condition, treatment and required nursing procedures to determine which supplies are needed.

## PLANNING

- Determine which supplies must be brought to the room so as to avoid putting on and removing the isolation gown unnecessarily.

### Equipment

According to the required nursing procedures, ensure that supplies are readily available.

1. Isolation gown of the proper size
2. Coat rack
3. Alcohol-based hand rub

# 技能操作 4 穿脱隔离衣法

护士护理传染病人时需穿隔离衣以保护病人和医务人员,避免交叉感染。

二维码 4-2

## 目的

- 保护医务人员和病人不受潜在感染性物质的污染(如血液、其他体液)。

## 评估

- 评估病人病情、治疗及护理操作要求以确定所需用物。

## 计划

- 备齐所需用物以免不必要的穿脱隔离衣。

### 用物准备

根据护理操作要求,备齐用物。

1.大小合适的隔离衣
2.挂衣架
3.速干手消毒剂

# IMPLEMENTATION

## Donning on an isolation gown

### Preparation

1. Trim fingernails. Remove or secure all loose items, such as name tags, watches and jewelry. **Rationale:** *It is difficult to disinfect once contaminated and disinfection easily makes them damaged.*

2. Roll the sleeves above the elbows (to the middle part of forearms in winter).

### Procedure

1. Perform hand hygiene, and put on a mask.

2. Pick up an isolation gown from the coat rack by holding the collar with one hand (if it has been used, the collar and the inside of the gown are considered clean). Hold each end of the collar with one hand. Unfold the gown in front of you with the inside of the gown facing you (see Figure 4-1).

# 实施

## 穿隔离衣法

### 准备

1. 修剪指甲，取下或保护好易掉落的物品，如胸牌、手表及饰物。**依据：**这些物品一旦被污染很难消毒，而且消毒易使这些物品受损。

2. 卷袖过肘（冬天至前臂中部）。

### 操作步骤

1. 洗手，戴口罩。

2. 手持衣领从挂衣架上取下隔离衣（如隔离衣已被穿过，其衣领和内面视为清洁面）。双手分别握住衣领两端，内面朝向自己展开隔离衣（见图4-1）。

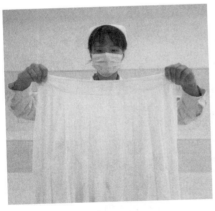

Figure 4-1　Letting the inside of the gown face you

图 4-1　隔离衣内面朝向自己

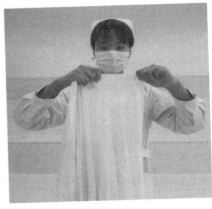

Figure 4-2　Moving one hand towards the other end of the collar

图 4-2　一手将衣领折向另一端

3. Move one hand towards the other end of the collar (see Figure 4-2). Put the free hand and arm in one sleeve while holding the collar and pulling up the sleeve with the other hand (see Figure 4-3). Hold the collar with the hand of the gowned arm and then insert the other hand and arm into the free sleeve (see Figure 4-4).

3. 一手慢慢将领子折向另一端握住（见图4-2），另一手伸入一侧袖内，持衣领的手向上拉，将衣袖穿好（见图4-3）。换手持衣领，同法穿好另一袖（见图4-4）。

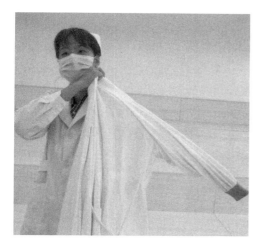

Figure 4-3    Putting the free hand and arm in one sleeve

图 4-3    一手伸入一侧衣袖内

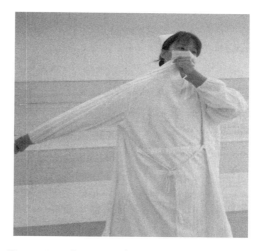

Figure 4-4    Inserting the other hand and arm into the free sleeve

图 4-4    另一手伸入衣袖

4. Button the collar while tilting the head and elbows backwards as much as possible to avoid contaminating your head and face (the hands are still considered clean) (see Figure 4-5).

4. 头尽量后仰,肘部向外展,扣好衣领,避免污染头面部(此时手仍然清洁)(见图 4-5)。

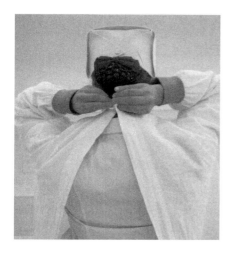

Figure 4-5    Buttoning the collar

图 4-5    扣领扣

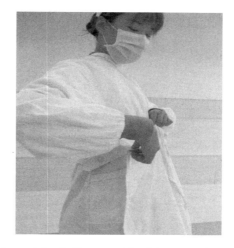

Figure 4-6    Pulling one side of the gown forward gradualy till reaching the edge

图 4-6    将隔离衣一边逐渐向前拉至触及衣边

5. Gradually pull one side of the gown forward (about 5cm below waist) and hold it when you reach the edge (the hands are contaminated now) (see Fig-

5. 将隔离衣一边(约在腰下5cm处)逐渐向前拉,见到衣边捏住(此时手已污染)(见图 4-6),

ure 4-6). Pull the other side of the gown forward in the same way. Make the gown edges parallel (see Figure 4-7) and overlap the gown at the back as much as possible (see Figure 4-8 (a), (b)), or roll the gown at the back (see Figure 4-9), and tie the waist strings in front (see Figure 4-10). Make sure that your hands do not touch the inside of the gown.

同法捏住另一侧衣边。两手在背后将衣襟边缘对齐（见图 4-7），向一侧折叠（见图 4-8（a），（b））或卷紧（见图 4-9），将腰带在腰前打一活结（见图 4-10），手勿触及隔离衣内面。

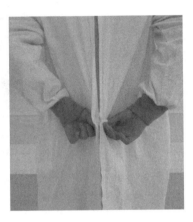

Figure 4-7  Making the gown edges parallel at the back

图 4-7  在背后将两衣边边缘对齐

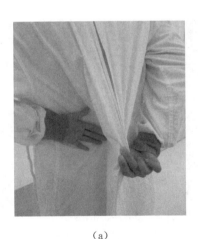

（a）

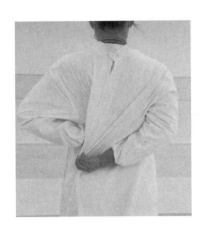

（b）

Figure 4-8  Overlapping the gown

图 4-8  向一侧折叠

### Removing an isolation gown

1. Untie the strings and make a slipnot in front.

2. Pull up the sleeves (to the middle part of forearms in winter) without exposing uniform sleeves (see Figure 4-11).

### 脱隔离衣法

1. 解开腰带，在前面打一活结。

2. 拉高衣袖（冬天拉至前臂中部），勿暴露工作服袖子（见图 4-11）。

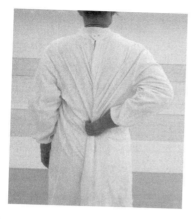

Figure 4-9　Rolling the gown at the back

图 4-9　向一侧卷起

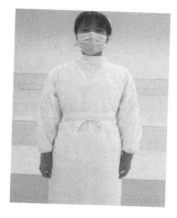

Figure 4-10　Tying the waist strings in front (making a bow)

图 4-10　腰带在前面打一活结

3. Perform hand hygiene, disinfecting both hands with alcohol-based hand rub.

4. Unbutton the collar. Pull one sleeve down to cover the hand by holding the inside of the sleeve with the other hand (see Figure 4-12). **Rationale：** *Clean hands can only touch the clean side of the gown.* Pull the other sleeve down by holding the outer surface of the sleeve with the gown-covered hand (see Figure 4-13). Avoid touching soiled side of the gown with your hands.

3. 按七步洗手法,用速干手消毒剂消毒双手。

4. 解开衣领,一手伸入另一侧袖口内拉下衣袖过手(遮住手)(见图 4-12)。**依据:**清洁的手只能触及隔离衣清洁面。再用衣袖遮住的手握住另一衣袖外面拉下袖子(见图 4-13),手勿触及隔离衣污染面。

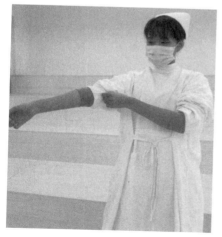

Figure 4-11　Making a slipknot in front, pulling up the sleeves

图 4-11　腰带在前面打一活结,拉高衣袖

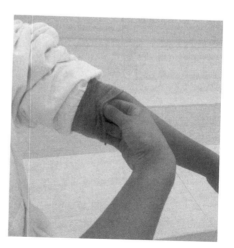

Figure 4-12　Pulling one sleeve down by holding the inside of the sleeve with the other hand

图 4-12　捏住对侧袖口内面拉下衣袖

5. Pull out both hands from the sleeves (see Figure 4-14).

6. If the gown will be used again, hold the collar of the gown with both hands (see Figure 4-15) and make the two sides of the gown parallel. Hang it on the rack (see Figure 4-16). **Rationale**: *Turn the inside of the gown outwards if it is to be hung in a half-contaminated area. Keep the outside of the gown outwards if it is to be hung in a contaminated area.*

5．双臂逐渐退出（见图 4-14）。

6．如隔离衣仍需使用，双手持衣领（见图 4-15），使两侧衣襟对齐挂于衣架上（见图 4-16）。**依据**：如挂在半污染区或清洁区，将隔离衣的内面向外；如挂在污染区则将衣服外面向外。

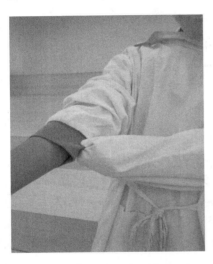

Figure 4-13　Pulling the other sleeve down by holding the outer surface of the sleeve with the gown-covered hand

图 4-13　用衣袖遮住的手握住另一衣袖的外面拉下袖子

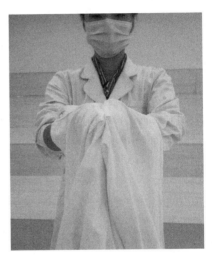

Figure 4-14　Pulling out both hands

图 4-14　双手退出衣袖

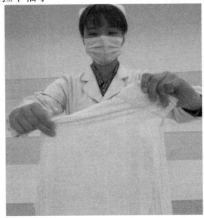

Figure 4-15　Holding the inside of the collar

图 4-15　手持衣领内面

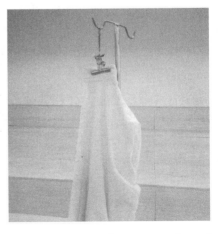

Figure 4-16　Hanging the gown on the rack

图 4-16　隔离衣挂在衣钩上

7. If it will not be used again, roll up the gown with the inner side and discard it in an appropriate container.

8. Perform hand hygiene.

## EVALUATION

• Ensure that an adequate supply of equipment is available for next use.

7. 不再穿的隔离衣将其内面向外卷起放于合适的置物袋内。

8. 洗手。

## 评价

• 确认下次操作用物已备齐。

## Words and Expressions

appropriate *adj.* 适当的,合适的
cross-infection（医）交叉感染
discard *vt.* 丢弃,抛弃
　（前缀 dis- 表示"不,相反或相对,分离"）
disinfect *vt.* 给……消毒
elbow *n.* 肘部
gown *n.* 长外衣,(尤指在医院穿的)外罩
isolate *vt.* (使)隔离,脱离

isolation *n.* 隔离,隔离状态
name tag 胸牌
parallel *adj.* 平行的
rack *n.* 架子,支架
tag *n.* 标签,标牌
tilt *v.* (使)倾斜,倾侧
slipknot *n.* 活结
untie *vt.* 解开……结,打开

# SKILL 5　Making Beds

# 技能操作5 铺床法

Nurses need to prepare hospital beds in different ways for specific purposes. Regardless of what purpose the bed is to be prepared for, nurses should pay attention to the following points.

医院护士需根据不同目的以不同的铺床法准备病床，操作时应注意以下事项。

二维码 5-1

二维码 5-2

## CLINICAL ALERTS

1. Wash hands thoroughly after handling a patient's bed linen. Linens that has been soiled by excretions and secretions harbor microorganisms which can be transmitted to others directly or indirectly through the nurses' hands or uniforms.

2. Get all linens ready before starting to strip the bed to avoid unnecessary trips to the linen supply area.

3. When stripping or making a beds, save time and energy by stripping or making one side before working on the other side.

4. Linens used by one patient should never (even momentarily) be placed on another patient's bed. **Rationale**: *This prevents cross-contamination via soiled linens.*

5. Roll soiled linens from the head of the bed to the end of the bed. Do not shake the soiled linens in the air so as to avoid disseminating pathogenic microorganisms that they contain.

6. Hold the soiled linens away from your uniform.

## 注意事项

1. 接触病人的被服后应彻底洗手。被排泄物和分泌物玷污的被服携带大量微生物，可直接或间接通过护士的双手或工作服传播给他人。

2. 操作前备齐用物以免不必要的走动。

3. 拆除床单或铺床时，应完成一侧再转至另一侧以省时省力。

4. 勿将病人被服放于其他病床上（即使是暂时放置）。**依据**: 防止交叉感染。

5. 污被服应从床头卷至床尾。勿抖动污被服，以免向外播散病原微生物。

6. 勿将污被服靠近自身工作服。

# 5-1　Making an Unoccupied Closed Bed

## PURPOSE

• To prepare a neat, wrinkle-free and comfortable bed for the patient.

## ASSESSMENT

1. Ensure that all linens are available and folded as required.

2. Check whether the quilt is suitable for the season.

3. Check if any patients in the room are receiving treatment or having meal, and if the ward is clean and well ventilated.

4. Check any bed damage.

## PLANNING

### Equipment

1. Bottom sheet

2. Cotton quilt/duvet

3. Cotton quilt cover/duvet cover

4. Pillow

5. Pillowcase

6. Additional equipment for the postoperative bed:

(1) 2 waterproof drawsheets, 2 linen drawsheets.

(2) Treatment tray: mouth opener, spatula, tongue forceps, air tubing, dental pad, tissue forceps, oxygen delivery device and connecting tube, suction catheters and connecting tube, kidney dish, sterile gauze, clean bowl, swabs.

(3) Oxygen supply, suction machine or wall suction outlet, ECG monitor, sphygmomanometer, stethoscope, flashlight, hot water bag with cover if necessary.

# 5-1　铺备用床法

## 目的

• 为病人准备整洁、无皱褶、舒适的床单位。

## 评估

1. 确定铺床所需用物已备齐,并按要求折叠。

2. 查看盖被是否适合当季气温。

3. 查看病室内有无病人正在治疗或进餐,病室是否清洁,通风是否良好。

4. 检查病床有无损坏。

## 计划

### 用物准备

1. 底单(大单)

2. 棉胎/羽绒被

3. 棉胎被套/羽绒被套

4. 枕芯

5. 枕套

6. 麻醉床另备:

(1)橡胶中单2块,中单2块。

(2)治疗盘内备:张口器、压舌板、拉舌钳、通气导管、牙垫、镊子、吸氧用具及连接管、吸痰管及连接管、弯盘、无菌纱布、清洁碗、棉签。

(3)供氧装置、负压吸引器或中心负压吸引管路、心电监护仪、血压计、听诊器、手电筒,必要时备热水袋及布套。

## IMPLEMENTATION

### Procedure

1. Perform hand hygiene, and put on a mask.

2. Place the clean linens in the order that they are going to be used (from top to bottom: bottom sheet, quilt cover, cotton quilt, pillowcase, pillow) on a trolley and carry them to the bedside.

3. Move the bedside table and the chair away from the bed to facilitate the procedure.

4. Lock the wheel of the bed, and raise the bed to a comfortable working height (if necessary) to save energy.

5. Check the mattress. Grab the lugs, if present, and move the mattress up to the head of bed. Turn it over if necessary.

6. Spread the bottom sheet:

(1) Place the bottom sheet on the mattress, with its center fold in the middle of the bed (see Figure 5-1) and set aside sufficient length of the sheet to be tucked under the top of the mattress. Unfold it lengthwise and spread it over the mattress (see Figure 5-2). **Rationale**: *The top of the sheet needs to be well tucked under the mattress to remain securely in place, especially when the head of the bed is elevated.*

## 实施

### 操作步骤

1.洗手，戴口罩。

2.将清洁床单按操作顺序放于治疗车上（从上到下：大单、被套、棉胎、枕套、枕芯），携至病人床旁。

3.移开床旁桌和椅，便于操作。

4.有脚轮的床，锁住床脚轮，必要时摇床至合适的操作高度以节省体力。

5.检查床垫，抓住吊耳将床垫上移紧靠床头。必要时翻转。

6.铺大单：

（1）放大单于床垫上，大单中缝对齐床面纵中线（见图5-1），床头留出足够长度，纵向打开大单（见图 5-2）。**依据**：足够长的床头大单方可包住床垫，尤其当床头抬高时。

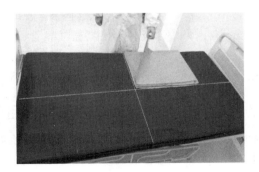

Figure 5-1　Placing the bottom sheet on the mattress, with its center fold in the middle of the bed

图5-1　放大单于床垫上，大单中缝对齐床面纵中线

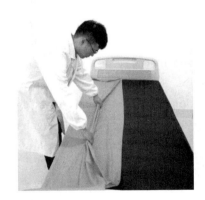

Figure 5-2　Spreading the bottom sheet lengthwise on the bed

图5-2　将大单纵向打开

（2）Tuck the top edge of the bottom sheet under the mattress and make the first envelope corner (an angle of 45°) near it, working from the head of the bed to the foot. Pull the sheet firmly towards the foot of the bed and make the second envelope corner (see Figure 5-3(a)-(f)). Move to the middle of the bed and tuck the side of the buttom sheet under the mattress. **Rationale**：*Completing one side of the bed at a time saves time and energy.*

（3）Move to the other side and secure the bottom sheet in the same manner. Firmly pull the remainder of the sheet so that there are no wrinkles. **Rationale**：*Wrinkles can cause discomfort for the patient and breakdown of skin.*

7. Cover the quilt：

（1）Place the quilt cover with its center fold in the middle of the bed (identical to the previous steps for the bottom sheet), and spread the quilt cover over the bottom sheet. The top edge of the quilt cover should be coincide with the top edge of the mattress.

（2）Open the end of the quilt cover by pulling the upper layer of the cover towards the head of the bed.

（3）Place the quilt (folded in 'S' shape) in the opening of the quilt cover. The bottom edge of the quilt should coincide with the end of the bed.

（4）Pull the quilt up to the closed end of the quilt cover and spread it. Fit the top corners of the quilt into the top corners of the quilt cover. Move to the end of the bed, pull the quilt cover smoothly and spread the end of quilt in the quilt cover. Adjust the quilt so that its corners fit into the corners of the quilt cover and the seams are straight. **Rationale**：*A smoothly fitting quilt cover is more comfortable than a wrinkled one.* Tie the strings of the quilt cover.

（5）Adjust the top edge of the quilt to coincide with the head of the bed.

（6）Fold the sides of the quilt to coincide with the edge of the bed. Fold the end of the quilt to coincide with the end of the bed (see Figure 5-4).

（2）将床头大单折入床垫下，"信封角"式铺好近侧床头角（45°角），移至床尾拉紧大单，同法铺好床尾角（见图5-3(a)～(f)），移至床中部，将大单中部边缘塞入床垫下。**依据**：铺好一侧再转至另一侧以省时省力。

（3）转至床对侧，同法铺对侧大单。在最后一角拉紧大单使其平紧。**依据**：床单皱褶会使病人不适及造成皮肤破损。

7. 套棉被：

（1）将被套中线与床中线对齐（同铺大单法），展开平铺于铺好的大单上，被套上端与床头平齐。

（2）将被套尾部开口端的上层打开。

（3）将"S"形折叠的棉胎放入被套尾端的开口处，被尾与床尾平齐。

（4）拉棉胎至被套头端并展开，两床头棉胎角对好被套角。转至床尾，拉平被套，将尾部棉胎展开平铺于被套内，充实被尾两角，对齐被缝。**依据**：四角充实的被子使病人舒适。系好被套系带。

（5）拉盖被上缘与床头平齐。

（6）两侧棉被边缘向内折叠和床沿平齐，床尾棉被向内折叠与床尾平齐（见图5-4）。

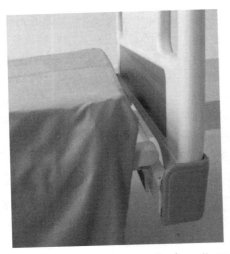

(a) Tucking the sheet firmly under the mattress

(a) 拉紧大单塞于床垫下

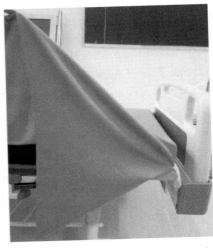

(b) Lifting the sheet so that it forms a triangle with the side edge of the bed

(b) 提起大单边缘，使大单与床缘呈三角形

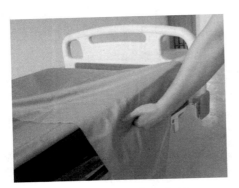

(c) Tucking the part of the sheet that hangs below the mattress under the mattress

(c) 垂于床垫下方的床单塞入床垫下

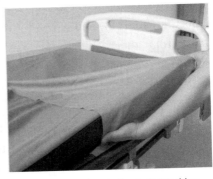

(d) Withdrawing the hand after tucking

(d) 撤出塞床单的手

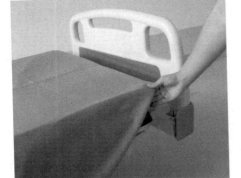

(e) Drooping the tip of the triangle down toward the floor

(e) 三角形的另一半大单垂于床缘

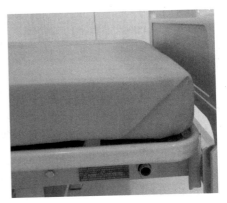

(f) Tucking the remainder of the sheet under the mattress

(f) 下垂的床单塞入床垫下

Figure 5-3　Making the corner of the bed

图 5-3　铺床角

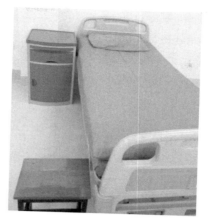

Figure 5-4　An unoccupied closed bed

图 5-4　备用床

8. Fit the pillow in a clean pillowcase:

（1）Hold the closed end of the pillowcase at the center with one hand. Gather up the open side of the pillowcase with its inside out. Hold the center of one short side of the pillow. Then pull the pillowcase over the pillow with the free hand（see Figure 5-5（a），(b)).

8. 套枕套：

（1）一手抓住清洁枕套封口端的中间，将枕套套于手上。用抓住枕套的手抓住枕芯一短边的中间，另一手拉枕套，套于枕芯外（见图 5-5(a)，(b)）。

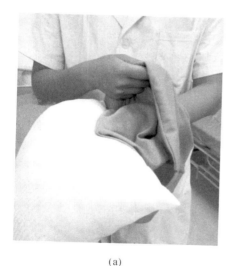

(a)

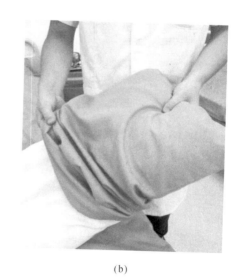

(b)

Figure 5-5　Putting a clean pillowcase on a pillow

图 5-5　套枕套

（2）Adjust the pillowcase so that the pillow fits into the corners of the pillowcase and the seams are straight. Place the pillow appropriately at the head of

（2）调整枕套使其四角充实，枕头缝对齐，放于床头中间，枕套开口端背门。

the bed with the closed end facing the door.

9. Move back the bedside table and chair so that they are available to the patient.

10. Return the bed to the low position.

11. Perform hand hygiene.

## 5-2　Making an Unoccupied Open Bed

An unoccupied open bed is prepared for a patient who temporarily leaves the bed. Generally, the quilt is folded back three or four times (different from an unoccupied closed bed), thus the term 'open bed'. This procedure makes it easier for the patient to get in (see Figure 5-6(a), (b)).

9. 移回床旁桌和椅，供病人使用。

10. 摇床至原来高度。

11. 洗手。

## 5-2　铺暂空床法

暂空床供暂时离床的病人使用。与备用床不同，暂空床是将棉被三折或四折折向床尾（"暂空床"的由来），便于病人躺卧（见图5-6(a), (b)）。

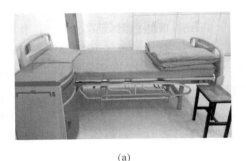
(a)

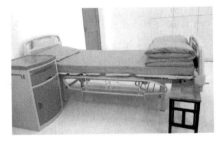
(b)

Figure 5-6　An unoccupied open bed

图 5-6　暂空床

## 5-3　Making a Surgical Bed

A surgical bed is used for the patient who is having surgery and will return to the bed for postoperative care. Nurses should make the bed as soon as the patient goes to surgery.

### IMPLEMENTATION

Procedure

1. Perform hand hygiene, and put on a mask.

2. Strip the bed.

3. Spread the bottom sheet and the waterproof drawsheet：

## 5-3　铺麻醉床法

麻醉床用于接收和护理麻醉手术后的病人，护士应在病人送去手术室后即刻铺好麻醉床。

### 实施

操作实施

1. 洗手，戴口罩。

2. 拆除污被服。

3. 铺大单和橡胶单：

(1) Spread the bottom sheet at one side of the bed as for an unoccupied closed bed.

(2) Put the waterproof drawsheet on the bed with the center fold at the center of the bed and the top edge 45 to 50 cm away from the head of the bed. Fanfold the uppermost half at the center, or the far edge, of the bed. Put the cloth drawsheet over the waterproof sheet in the same way, then tuck them under the mattress.

(3) According to the operation site or type of anesthesia, place the other waterproof drawsheet and the other cloth drawsheet in sequence at the head (top edge of the drawsheets should coincide with the head of the bed) or end (bottom edge of the drawsheets should coincide with the end of the bed) of the bed, then tuck them under the mattress.

(4) Move to the other side and secure the bottom linen as for an unoccupied closed bed.

(5) Pull the drawsheets firmly and tuck them under the mattress.

4. Cover the quilt as for an unoccupied closed bed.

5. Fanfold the quilt on the side of the bed away from the door. **Rationale**: *This facilitates the patient's transfer into the bed.*

6. Fit the pillow with a clean pillowcase as you would for an unoccupied bed, but put the pillow in an upright position at the head of bed.

7. Move back the bedside table.

8. Move the chair at the fanfolded quilt side of the bed to facilitate transferring the patient (see Figure 5-7).

9. Leave the bed in the high position with the side rails down. **Rationale**: *The high position facilitates the transfer of the patient.* Lock the wheels of the bed. **Rationale**: *Locking the wheels keeps the bed from rolling when the patient is transferred from the trolley to the bed.*

10. Perform hand hygiene.

11. Leave the treatment tray on the bedside table.

（1）按备用床法铺好近侧大单。

（2）铺橡胶单，中线与床中线对齐，上缘距床头 45～50 cm，扇形折叠上层橡胶单于床中线或至对侧，同法铺中单在橡胶单上，床缘部分一并塞入床垫下。

（3）根据手术部位或麻醉类型，依次铺另一橡胶单和中单于床头（橡胶单和中单上缘与床头平齐）或床尾（橡胶单和中单下缘与床尾平齐），床缘部分一并塞入床垫下。

（4）转至对侧，按备用床法铺好大单。

（5）拉紧橡胶单和中单，塞入床垫下。

4. 按备用床法套好棉被。

5. 将盖被扇形折叠到背门一侧。**依据**：利于搬运病人。

6. 按备用床法套好枕头，横立于床头。

7. 移回床旁桌。

8. 将椅子放于折叠被同侧以利于搬运（见图5-7）。

9. 保持床在高位，放下床栏。**依据**：床高利于搬运。固定床脚轮。**依据**：以免搬运病人时脚轮滚动。

10. 洗手。

11. 将麻醉护理盘放于床旁桌上。

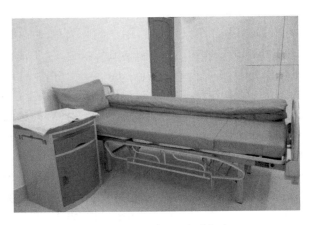

Figure 5-7　A surgical bed

图 5-7　麻醉床

## EVALUATION

1. The bed is neat，wrinkle-free and comfortable.

2. The call bell is accessible to the patient.

3. All needed equipment is available and functioning well.

## 评价

1. 床铺平紧、无皱褶、舒适。

2. 呼叫铃方便取用。

3. 所需用物已备齐，性能良好。

# Words and Expressions

anaesthesia/anesthesia *n.* 麻醉

anaesthetic *adj.* 麻醉的；*n.* 麻醉剂，麻醉药

anaesthetic/postoperative/surgical bed 麻醉床

bottom drawsheet 底单，大单

call bell 呼叫铃，电铃

catheter *n.* 导管(如导尿管)

cross-contamination (病菌的)交叉污染

delivery *n.* 递送，分娩

dental *adj.* 牙科的，牙齿的

dental pad 牙垫

device *n.* 装置，仪器，设备

drawsheet *n.* (住院病人用的)垫单

duvet *n.* 羽绒被

electrocardiograph (ECG) *n.* 心电图

　(前缀 electro- 表示"电的")

firmly *adv.* 坚定地，坚固地

flashlight *n.* 手电筒

kidney *n.* 肾

kidney dish/bowl 弯盘

length *n.* 长度，长

lengthwise *adv.* 纵向，纵长

linen/cloth drawsheet 中单

lug *n.* 手柄，把手

mattress *n.* 床垫

momentarily *adv.* 短暂地，片刻地

oxygen *n.* 氧气，氧

oxygen delivery device 吸氧用具

pillowcase *n.* 枕套

postoperative *adj.* 手术后的

　(前缀 post- 表示"后，以后")

seam *n.* 线缝，接缝

side rails/cot sides/safety sides 床档，床栏

spatula/tongue blade/tongue depressor *n.*
压舌板

sphygmomanometer/blood pressure meter
*n.* 血压计

stethoscope *n.* 听诊器

strip *vt.* 除去,剥去(一层)

suction *n.* 吸,抽吸,吸出

surgery *n.* 外科学,外科手术

surgical *adj.* 外科的,外科手术的

temporarily *adv.* 临时地,短暂地

tongue forceps 拉舌钳

tuck *vt.* (把衣服、纸张等的边缘)塞进,折起

unoccupied *adj.* 空着的,闲置的

unoccupied closed bed 备用床

unoccupied open bed 暂空床

uppermost *adj.* 最上面的,最高的

ventilate *vt.* 使(房间、建筑物等)通风,使
通气

ventilation *n.* 通风,通气

waterproof *adj.* 不透水的,防水的

waterproof/rubber drawsheet 防水单,橡
胶单

wrinkle *n.* 皱褶,皱纹

# SKILL 6　Changing an Occupied Bed

Patients may not be able to get out of the bed because of various reasons, such as weakness, unconsciousness, the consequences of diseases, traction or other therapies. Nurses need to change the sheets while the bed is occupied. This process can be strenuous for the person occupying the bed, so make sure your supplies are ready beforehand to streamline the process as much as possible.

二维码 6-1

## CLINICAL ALERTS

1. Never move or position a patient in a manner that is contraindicated in the patient with his/her disease. If needed, get help to ensure safety.

2. Move the patient gently and with caution. Rough handling can cause discomfort and bruises.

3. Explain to the patient what you are going to do before you do it. Use terms that the patient can understand.

4. Assess the patient and meet the patient's needs while making the bed.

5. Changing an occupied bed easily disturbs the patient, so be as considerate as possible to try to save the patient's energy.

6. Adhere to safe moving and handling techniques so that you don't cause harm to the patient and yourself.

## PURPOSES

1. To provide a smooth, wrinkle-free bed, thus minimizing skin irritation.

2. To promote patient's comfort.

# 技能操作6　卧床病人更换床单法

病人可能因极度虚弱、意识不清、疾病、牵引或其他治疗等原因不能下床，护士也需为其更换床单。为卧床病人更换床单时易耗费病人体力，操作前必须备齐用物，尽可能使操作顺利进行。

二维码 6-2

## 注意事项

1. 移动或安置病人体位时切勿影响病情。

2. 小心移动病人，动作粗暴将引起病人不适和皮肤擦伤。

3. 操作前运用通俗语言向病人解释操作内容。

4. 利用铺床时间评估病人，满足其需求。

5. 更换床单容易干扰病人，操作时尽量为病人着想以保存其体力。

6. 运用安全移动技术，避免对病人和自身造成伤害。

## 目的

1. 提供平整、无皱褶的床单位以减少皮肤刺激。

2. 促进病人舒适。

## ASSESSMENT

1. Determine specific precautions for moving and positioning the patient.

2. Check if there is of incontinence or excessive drainage to determine if there is need for protective waterproof pads.

3. Assess skin condition and determine if there is need for special mattress.

4. Check if any patients are receiving treatment or having meals in the room, and if the ward is clean and well ventilated.

5. Determine whether an assistant is needed; if so, seek help.

## PLANNING

### Equipment

1. Bottom sheet
2. Cloth/linen drawsheet
3. Pillowcase
4. Bed brush with disposable moist brush cover

## IMPLEMENTATION

### Procedure

1. Perform hand hygiene, and put on a mask.

2. Put the bed brush and clean linens in the order that they are going to be used (from top to bottom: bottom sheet, linen drawsheet, pillowcase) on a trolley and carry them to the bedside.

3. Explain the procedure to the patient and promote cooperation.

4. Move away the bedside table and the chair from the bed. **Rationale**: *This facilitates the procedure.*

5. Raise the bed to a comfortable working height (if possible). **Rationale**: *This avoids over bending the lower back to reduce risk of injury to nurses.*

6. Remove any equipment attached to the bed linen.

7. Change the bottom sheet and the drawsheet:

## 评估

1. 移动和安置病人时应采取的防护措施。

2. 有无大小便失禁或引流液量以确定是否需要防护垫。

3. 皮肤情况,是否需要特殊床垫。

4. 病房内是否有病人正在治疗或进餐,病室是否清洁,通风是否良好。

5. 是否需要助手,必要时寻求帮助。

## 计划

### 用物准备

1. 大单
2. 中单
3. 枕套
4. 床刷(套有一次性微湿床刷套)

## 实施

### 操作步骤

1. 洗手,戴口罩。

2. 将床刷及清洁床单按使用顺序放于治疗车上(从上到下:大单、中单、枕套),携至病人床旁。

3. 向病人解释,取得配合。

4. 移开床旁桌和椅。**依据**: 便于操作。

5. 如条件允许,摇床至舒适的操作高度。**依据**:避免过度弯腰以降低护士腰部受伤的风险。

6. 移开床单上的用物。

7. 更换大单及中单:

（1）If possible，raise the side rail so that the patient will turn around himself. If there is none，have another nurse support the patient at the edge of the bed. **Rationale：** *This protects the patient from falling off the bed.*

（2）Adjust the pillow. Help the patient to turn away from your side.

（3）Loosen all at once：the bottom sheet，the rubber drawsheet and the linen drawsheet at the near side of the bed.

（4）Tuck the dirty linen drawsheet under the patient. Wipe off debris on the rubber drawsheet with a bed brush. Place the rubber drawsheet on the patient.

（5）Tuck the dirty bottom sheet at the middle of the bed and under the patient as possible（see Figure 6-1）. **Rationale：** *It leaves the near half of the bed free to be changed.* Clean the mattress with the bed brush.

（6）Place the clean bottom sheet on the mattress，with its center fold in the middle of the bed（see Figure 6-2(a)，(b)）. Tuck lengthwise the uppermost half of the bottom sheet under the patient as possible. Make the envelop corners at the near side and tuck the sheet under the mattress as for an unoccupied closed bed.

（1）有床栏者拉起对侧床栏；如无床栏，另一护士须在床旁扶住病人。**依据：** 避免病人坠床。

（2）移枕头至对侧，协助病人背向护士侧卧。

（3）将近侧大单、橡胶单及中单一起松开。

（4）卷污中单于病人身下，用床刷扫净橡胶单上的碎屑，搭于病人身上。

（5）卷污大单于床中间，尽可能塞入病人身下（见图 6-1）。**依据：** 使近侧床垫留出足够空间铺大单。用床刷扫净床垫。

（6）铺清洁大单于床垫上，大单中缝与床中线对齐（见图 6-2(a)，(b)）。纵向卷起上层大单塞入病人身下，按备用床法铺好近侧床角和大单。

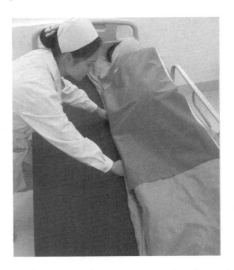

Figure 6-1　Tucking the dirty bottom linen under the patient as possible

图 6-1　污大单尽可能塞入病人身下

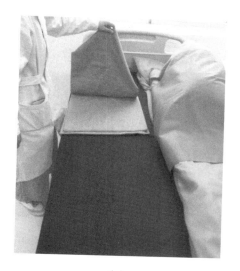
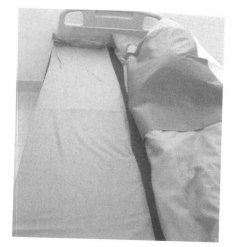

(a)                                                                                  (b)

Figure 6-2    Placing a clean bottom sheet on half of the bed

图 6-2   铺近侧清洁大单

　　(7) Reposition the rubber drawsheet，and place the clean linen drawsheet over the rubber drawsheet (see Figure 6-3). The middle of the drawsheets should coincide with the middle of the bed. Tuck the uppermost half of the clean linen drawsheet lengthwise at the middle of the bed and tuck the near side of both drawsheets under the mattress.

　　（7）放平橡胶单，将清洁中单的中缝与床中线对齐铺在橡胶单上（见图 6-3），卷起远侧一半清洁中单塞于病人身下，将近侧橡胶单和中单一起塞入床垫下。

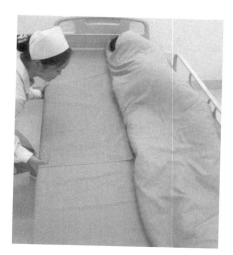

Figure 6-3    Placing a clean linen drawsheet on the rubber drawsheet

图 6-3   铺清洁中单于橡胶单上

(8) Assist the patient to lie on his/her back.

(9) Raise the side rail.

(10) Move to the other side of the bed and lower the side rail.

(11) Move the pillow to the clean side for the patient to use. Assist the patient to roll to the clean side of the bed.

(12) Loosen the bottom sheet and two drawsheets at once. Remove the soiled linen drawsheet by folding it (the soiled side turned in) and roll it towards the end of the bed. Wipe off debris on the rubber drawsheet with the bed brush. Place the rubber drawsheet on the patient.

(13) Carefully remove used linens and place them on the lower layer of the trolley. Clean the mattress with the bed brush from the head to the end of the bed.

(14) Unfold the bottom sheet and pull it firmly with both hands, so that it becomes smooth. Make the rest corners and tuck the rest of the bottom sheet under the mattress. Reposition the rubber drawsheet. Pull out the linen drawsheet with both hands. Tuck the rest of the drawsheets under the mattress.

8. Assist the patient to lie flat in the middle of the bed.

9. Change the pillowcase and place the pillow under the patient's head.

10. Smooth down his/her clothes. Assist him/her to a comfortable position.

11. Tuck the patient in:

(1) Spread the quilt over the patient at one side. Fold the side edge of the quilt along the edge of the bed. Fold the end of the quilt along the end of the bed.

(2) Repeat the action on the other side of the bed.

12. Return the bedside table and the chair to their place.

13. Ensure a safe environment for the patient:

(1) Place the bed in the low position. Raise the side rails if needed.

（8）协助病人平卧。

（9）拉起近侧床栏。

（10）转至对侧,放下床栏。

（11）移枕头于清洁侧,协助病人翻身侧卧于已铺好的一侧。

（12）将大单、橡胶单及中单一起松开,污中单污面向内卷起放于床尾,用床刷扫净橡胶单上的碎屑,搭于病人身上。

（13）轻轻将污大单卷起撤出,和污中单一起放于推车下层,从床头至床尾扫净床垫。

（14）拉出大单,双手用力将其拉紧,铺好两角。将边缘部分床单塞入床垫下。放平橡胶单,双手拉出中单,将两单一起塞入床垫下。

8. 协助病人平卧于床中间。

9. 更换枕套,放于病人头下。

10. 整理病人衣服,协助躺卧舒适。

11. 整理盖被:

（1）展开近侧盖被,被缘向内折与床沿齐,床尾盖被向内折叠与床尾平齐。

（2）转至对侧同法整理好盖被。

12. 移回床旁桌、椅。

13. 保证病人安全:

（1）将床摇低。必要时拉起床栏。

(2) Place the call bell and other items used by the patient in close proximity.

14. Provide appropriate instructions.

15. Perform hand hygiene.

## EVALUATION

• Conduct appropriate nursing interventions, such as checking patient's comfort and safety, patency of all drainage tubes and patient's access to the call bell to summon help when needed.

（2）将呼叫铃及其他用物放于病人易取之处。

14. 交代注意事项。

15. 洗手。

## 评价

• 实施合适的护理，如检查病人是否舒适、安全，引流管是否通畅，呼叫铃是否方便取用。

## Words and Expressions

attach *vt.* 把……固定，把……附（在……上）

bruise *n.* 青肿，瘀伤；*vt.* 撞伤，擦伤

caution *n.* 小心，谨慎

conscious *adj.* 神志清醒的，意识到的

consciousness *n.* 意识，知觉

contraindicate *vt.* 禁忌（某种药物或疗法）

（前缀 contra- 表示"反对，相反"）

contraindication *n.*（对某种药物或疗效）禁忌

debris *n.* 碎片，破片

disposable *adj.* 一次性的

disturb *vt.* 打扰，妨碍；*vi.* 打扰，妨碍

drain *vi.* 排空；*vt.* 使流出，流走

drainage *n.* 排水，放水

excessive *adj.* 过分的，过度的

incontinence *n.* 失禁，不能自制

（前缀 in- 表示"不，无，非，在……内"）

incontinent *adj.* 失禁的

intervention *n.* 干预，介入

meet the patient's needs 满足病人的需求

patency *n.* 开放，未闭

patent *adj.* 开放的，未闭的

precaution *n.* 预防措施，防备

（前缀 pre- 表示"先于，在……之前"）

reposition *vt.* 使复位，改变……的位置

streamline *v.* 使……效率更高

strenuous *adj.* 费力的，繁重的，艰苦的

summon *vt.* 召唤，请求

unconscious *adj.* 无意识的，昏迷的

unconsciousness *n.* 昏迷，无知觉状态

wipe off 擦干净，抹掉

# SKILL 7　Moving a Patient Up in Bed

Patients in the Fowler's position are likely to slide down the bed. Patients may have difficulty moving up in the bed independently because of illness or treatment limitations. According to patients' ability to move and their health conditions, there should be enough staff attending the procedure to avoid injuring themselves and patients.

二维码 7-1

## PURPOSE

● To assist patients who have slid down from the Fowler's position and move them up in bed to maintain their comfort and safety.

## ASSESSMENT

1. Assess the patient's physical ability to assist with the move (presence of paralysis, muscle strength).

2. Assess the patient's ability to understand instructions and willingness to participate.

3. Assess the patient's weight, condition, treatment. Identify presence of pain and need for analgesic or other pain relief measures.

4. Assess if there is need for assistance and auxiliary equipment.

## PLANNING

1. Determine the number of personnel and type of equipment needed to safely perform the positional change in order to prevent injury to staff and the patient.

2. Ensure that the patient understands instructions.

# 技能操作 7　协助病人移向床头法

病人取半坐卧位容易滑向床尾。由于疾病或治疗的限制，病人可能难以自行移向床头。护士应根据病人的移动能力和健康状况安排足够人员参与移动，以免自身和病人受伤。

二维码 7-2

## 目的

● 协助半坐卧位滑向床尾的病人移向床头，维持病人舒适及安全。

## 评估

1. 病人是否有移动能力（有无偏瘫、肌力状况）。

2. 病人理解指令的能力及合作意愿。

3. 病人体重、病情、治疗情况，有无疼痛，是否需要止痛剂或其他缓解疼痛的措施。

4. 是否需要助手及辅助器械。

## 计划

1. 确定操作所需人数和用物，防止自身和病人受伤。

2. 确定病人能理解指令。

## Equipment

- Assistive devices if needed

## IMPLEMENTATION

### Preparation

Check：

1. Any impediments to movement（such as an intravenous infusion or an indwelling urinary catheter）. Place them appropriately if necessary.

2. Medications that the patient is receiving, because certain medications may hamper movement or alertness of the patient.

3. Usually two nurses or nursing assistants are required to move a patient in a bed. **Rationale**：*Moving a patient is not a one-person task. During any patient handling, if the patient's weight is more than 16 kg, the patient should be considered fully dependent and assistive devices should be used, and more than two nurses should attend the procedure to reduce risk of injury to themselves.*

### Procedure

1. Before performing the procedure, verify the patient's identity. Introduce yourself and explain to the patient what you are going to do, why it is necessary, and how they can participate.

2. Protect the patient's privacy.

3. Perform hand hygiene.

4. Adjust the bed's and the patient's position：

（1）Lock the wheels of the bed. Adjust the head of the bed to a flat position or as low as the patient can tolerate. **Rationale**：*Save nurses' energy and prevent back strain.*

（2）Raise the side rail across from you.

（3）Remove all pillows and place one against the headboard. **Rationale**：*The pillow protects the patient's head from inadvertent injury against the top of the bed during the upward move.* Fanfold the quilt to the end of the bed as for an unoccupied open bed if necessary.

5. For the patient who is able to move up with-

## 用物准备

- 必要时准备辅助器械

## 实施

### 准备

确定：

1. 是否有影响移动病人的障碍（如静脉输液管或留置导尿管），必要时先妥善安置。

2. 病人用药情况。因某些药物会影响病人活动度或机敏度。

3. 一般需要两人。**依据**：移动病人通常不应由一人完成。如病人体重超过 16 kg，应属于完全依赖型，搬移时应使用辅助器械或由两人以上搬移，以降低护士受伤的风险。

### 操作步骤

1. 操作前自我介绍并确认病人，向病人解释操作内容、目的和配合方法。

2. 保护病人隐私。

3. 洗手。

4. 调整病床和病人的位置：

（1）固定床脚轮，摇平床头或摇至病人可耐受的高度。**依据**：节力并防止护士背部肌肉拉伤。

（2）拉起对侧床栏。

（3）移去全部枕头，将一个枕头横立于床头栏杆。**依据**：枕头横立可防止病人头部撞伤。必要时将盖被折到床尾铺成暂空床。

5. 对无须帮助、可自行移向

out assistance：

（1）Place the bed flat or the Trendelenburg's position (as tolerated by the patient). Assess if the patient is able to move without causing friction to the skin.

（2）Stand by and instruct the patient to move. Instruct the patient to hold the upper rails with both hands，flex the hips and knees and position the feet. Encourage him/her to straighten his/her back and move up with the arms pulling the rails and the feet treading on the bed. **Rationale**：*Flexing the hips and knees keeps the entire lower leg over the bed，preventing friction during movement，and ensures the use of the large muscle groups in the patient's legs，thus increasing the force of movement.*

6. For the patient who is partially able to assist：

（1）Ask the patient to hold the upper rails with both hands，and bend the hips and knees.

（2）Stand on one side of the bed，and place one hand under the patient's back and the other hand under the thighs. While looking at the patient, stand with feet apart，then lean forward with knees bent.

（3）Ask the patient to lift the head during the move to minimize friction.

（4）On the count of three, shift your weight to the front leg as the patient pulls the rails and treads on the bed so that the patient moves toward the head of the bed (see Figure 7-1).

床头的病人：

（1）将床头摇平或采用头低足高位（病人能耐受）。评估病人是否能移向床头且不擦伤皮肤。

（2）护士站在床边指导病人。嘱病人两手握住床头栏杆，屈髋屈膝，放好两脚位置。鼓励病人双手拉时两脚蹬床面，挺身上移。

**依据**：屈髋屈膝使双腿离开床面以避免移动时腿部与床面摩擦，并可利用腿部大肌群，增强移动力量。

6. 对有部分移动能力的病人：

（1）嘱病人两手握住床头栏杆，屈髋屈膝。

（2）护士站在床旁，一手托住病人肩背部，另一手托住大腿。面向床头，两脚分开，上身前倾，屈膝屈髋。

（3）嘱病人移动时抬头，以减少头部和床面的摩擦。

（4）当护士数到3时，嘱病人双手用力拉，双脚蹬床面，同时护士重心前移，协助病人移向床头（见图7-1）。

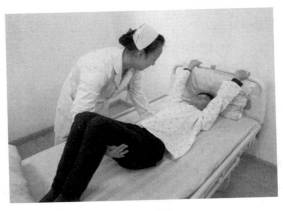

Figure 7-1　Helping the patient move up

图 7-1　帮助病人移向床头

7. For the patient who is unable to assist:

(1) Two nurses stand at each side of the bed next to the heaviest parts of the patient's body, which is usually the trunk and upper legs. Position themselves as previously described in step 6(1).

(2) Place the patient's arms across his/her abdomen. Ask the patient to lift the head during the move to minimize friction.

(3) Facing each other, the two nurses insert their hands under the patient's shoulders and buttocks, and interlock their fingers.

(4) When ready to move the patient, on the count of three, the two nurses will then move the patient towards the head of the bed.

8. Ensure the patient's comfort:

(1) Replace the pillow under the patient's head.

(2) Elevate the head of the bed and provide appropriate support devices for the patient.

9. Document all relevant information:

(1) Time of moving.

(2) Skin condition of pressure areas.

(3) Use of support devices.

(4) Ability of the patient to move.

(5) The reaction of the patient after moving (e. g., respiratory rate, pulse rate, anxiety, dizziness or discomfort).

## EVALUATION

1. The body mechanics is used during the move.

2. All catheters are placed properly and kept patent.

3. The patient is positioned safely and comfortably.

7.对无移动能力的病人：

(1)护士两人分别站于床的两侧,靠近病人躯干和大腿。站姿同步骤 6(1)。

(2)将病人两手交叉于腹部,嘱病人移动时抬头,减少头部和床面的摩擦。

(3)护士两人之间双手交叉,托住病人颈肩部和臀部。

(4)准备就绪,一护士数到 3 时,两人同时将病人抬起,移向床头。

8.保证病人舒适：

(1)放回枕头。

(2)摇高床头,安置病人。

9.记录：

(1)移向床头的时间。

(2)受压部位皮肤情况。

(3)使用的支撑物。

(4)病人移动能力。

(5)病人移动后的反应(如呼吸频率、脉率、情绪、头晕或不适情况)。

## 评价

1.移动病人时运用人体力学原理。

2.各导管安置妥当并保持通畅。

3.病人卧位安全、舒适。

# Words and Expressions

alert *vt.* 使警觉；*adj.* 警惕的,戒备的
alertness *n.* 警戒,机敏
（后缀-ness 表示"状态,性质"）

analgesic *n.* 镇痛剂,镇痛药
anxiety *n.* 焦虑,忧虑
assistive *adj.* 辅助的

buttock *n.* 半边臀部

dizziness *n.* 头晕,头昏眼花

flex *vt.* 屈曲

knee *n.* 膝,膝盖,膝关节

Fowler's position 半坐位(45°～60°角)

friction *n.* 摩擦,摩擦力

hamper *vt.* 妨碍,阻止,阻碍;*n.* 盛脏衣服
　的大篮子

hip *n.* 髋部,臀部

identify *vt.* 确认,鉴定

identity *n.* 身份,本身

impediment *n.* 障碍,阻碍

inadvertent *adj.* 不经意的,无意的

independently *adv.* 独立地,自主地

indwelling *adj.* 内在的,留置的

indwelling urinary catheter 留置导尿管

intravenous (IV) *adj.* 静脉内的
　(前缀 intra- 表示"在内,内部")

lean *vi.* 倾斜,倚靠

minimize *vt.* 使减少到最低限度

paralysis *n.* 麻痹,瘫痪

partially *adv.* 部分地,不完全地

participate *vi.* 参与,参加

privacy *n.* 隐私,秘密

pulse *n.* 脉搏,脉率

relevant *adj.* 紧密相关的,切题的

respiratory *adj.* 呼吸的

reverse *adj.* 反面的,相反的;*vt.* 颠倒,彻
　底转变

reverse Trendelenburg's position 头高足
　低位

slide *vi.* 滑行,滑动(过去式 slid,过去分词
　slid)

strength *n.* 力量,体力

thigh *n.* 大腿

Trendelenburg's position 头低足高位

trunk *n.* (人的)躯干

urinary *adj.* 尿的,尿路的
　(前缀 urin-/urino- 表示"尿")

verify *vt.* 核实,核准,查对

willingness *n.* 愿意,乐意

# SKILL 8　Turning a Patient to a Lateral Position in Bed

# 技能操作8　协助病人翻身侧卧法

Patients may have difficulty turning over in bed because of limitations caused by diseases or treatments. Nurses should help change their positions at regular intervals, and maintain a correct body alignment, so that undue stress is not placed on muscles and bones.

病人可能因疾病或治疗的限制难以自行翻身。护士应定期为其翻身,保持正确的卧床姿势,以免肌肉、骨骼受压过久。

二维码 8-1

二维码 8-2

## PURPOSES

1. To promote the patient's comfort.

2. To meet the needs for treatment or nursing care (e. g., when placing a bedpan beneath the patient, changing or tidying bed linens).

3. To prevent complications (e. g., pressure injuries) changing positions alternately.

## 目的

1. 改善病人的舒适度。

2. 满足治疗或护理需求(如放置便盆、整理或更换床单位)。

3. 变换卧位,预防多种并发症(如压力性损伤)。

## ASSESSMENT

1. Assess the patient's physical ability to assist with the move (presence of paralysis, muscle strength).

2. Assess the patient's ability to understand instructions and willingness to participate.

3. Assess the patient's weight, condition, treatment. Identify presence of pain and need for analgesic or other pain relief measures.

4. Assess if there is need for assistance and auxiliary equipment.

## 评估

1. 病人是否有移动能力(有无偏瘫、肌力状况)。

2. 病人理解指令的能力及合作意愿。

3. 病人体重、病情、治疗情况,有无疼痛,是否需要止痛剂或其他缓解疼痛的措施。

4. 是否需要助手及辅助器械。

## PLANNING

1. Determine the number of personnel and type of equipment needed to safely perform the positional

## 计划

1. 确定操作所需人数和用物,防止自身和病人受伤。

change in order to prevent injury to staff and the patient.

2. Ensure that the patient understands instructions.

## Equipment

- Pillows

## IMPLEMENTATION

### Preparation

Check：

1. Any impediments to turning over (such as an intravenous infusion or an indwelling urinary cathe-ter). Place them appropriately if necessary.

2. Medications the patient is receiving, because certain medications may hamper movement or alertness of the patient.

3. Usually two nurses or nursing assistants are required to turn over a patient in a bed. **Rationale**：*Turning over a patient is not a one-person task. During any patient handling，if the patient's weight is more than 16 kg，the patient should be considered fully dependent and assistive devices should be used，and more than two nurses should attend the procedure to reduce risk of injury to themselves.*

### Procedure

1. Prior to performing the procedure, introduce yourself and verify the patient's identity. Explain to the patient the procedure, purposes and how they can participate.

2. Protect the patient's privacy.

3. Perform hand hygiene.

4. Lock the wheels of the bed.

5. Adjust the head of the bed to a flat position or as low as the patient can tolerate if the patient is in a Fowler's position.

6. Raise the side rail which the patient will turn to.

7. Two nurses stand at the same side of the bed, place the patient's arms across his/her abdomen, and bend the knees. The nurse who is close to the patient's head places one hand on the patient's shoulder and the other on his/her lower back. At the

2. 确定病人能理解指令。

## 用物准备

- 枕头数个

## 实施

### 准备

确定：

1. 是否有影响病人翻身的障碍（如静脉输液管或留置导尿管），必要时先妥善安置。

2. 病人用药情况。因某些药物可影响病人的活动度或机敏度。

3. 一般需要两人。**依据**：翻动病人通常不应由一人完成。如病人体重超过 16 kg，应属于完全依赖型，搬移时应使用辅助器械或由两人以上搬移，以降低护士受伤的风险。

### 操作步骤

1. 操作前自我介绍并确认病人，向病人解释操作内容、目的和配合方法。

2. 保护病人隐私。

3. 洗手。

4. 固定床脚轮。

5. 如病人为半坐卧位，先摇平床头，或摇至病人能耐受的高度。

6. 拉起对侧床栏。

7. 两名护士站在病床同侧。将病人双手交叉于腹部，屈膝。靠近床头的护士托住病人颈肩和腰部，另一护士托住臀部和腘窝。

same time, the other nurse places one hand under the patient's hip and the other under knees.

8. Position yourself appropriately before performing the movement:

(1) Simultaneously lift the patient up, and move the patient to the near edge of the bed. **Rationale**: *This ensures that the patient will be positioned safely in the center of the bed after turning.*

(2) Place the patient's near arm across his/her chest and the opposite one beside the head with its elbow flexed. **Rationale**: *This prevents the arm from being pressed beneath the patient's body after turning.*

(3) Place the patient's near ankle across the other one.

9. Assist the patient to turn to the lateral position:

(1) The nurse who is close to the patient's head places her hands under the patient's shoulder and lower back. While the nurse who is close to the patient's feet places her hands under the patient's hip and knees.

(2) Turn the patient to the lateral position simultaneously. Position the patient at the center of the bed on his/her side.

10. Check the skin condition of pressure areas. Provide skin care if needed.

11. Position and support the arms and legs with pillows properly.

12. Place the call bell within the patient's reach.

13. Perform hand hygiene.

14. Record all relevant information:

(1) Time of turning and the positions before and after turning.

(2) Skin condition of pressure areas.

(3) Use of support devices.

(4) Ability of the patient to assist in moving and turning.

(5) The patient's response to turning (e. g., respiratory rate, pulse rate, anxiety, discomfort, dizziness).

8. 操作前护士站好位置：

（1）护士两人同时将病人抬起,移向近侧床边。**依据**:保证病人翻身后躺卧于床中间。

（2）将病人近侧手臂置于胸前,远侧手臂屈肘置于头侧。**依据**:避免翻身后手臂受压。

（3）将病人的近侧脚踝交叉置于对侧脚踝上。

9. 协助病人翻身侧卧：

（1）床头护士一手扶肩,一手扶腰；床尾护士一手扶臀,一手扶膝。

（2）两人动作一致轻推病人,使病人转向对侧,侧卧于床中间。

10. 检查受压部位皮肤情况,必要时进行皮肤护理。

11. 妥善安置并用软枕支撑病人手脚。

12. 将床头铃放于病人易取之处。

13. 洗手。

14. 记录：

（1）翻身时间,翻身前后体位。

（2）受压部位皮肤情况。

（3）支撑用物。

（4）病人移动和翻身的能力。

（5）翻身后的反应(如呼吸频率、脉率、情绪、不适和头晕情况)。

## EVALUATION

1. The body mechanics are used during the turn.

2. All catheters are placed properly and kept patent.

3. The patient is positioned safely and comfortably.

## 评价

1. 翻动病人时运用人体力学原理。

2. 各导管安置妥当并保持通畅。

3. 病人卧位安全、舒适。

# Words and Expressions

abdomen *n.* 腹(部)

abdominal *adj.* 腹部的

alignment *n.* 排成直线

alternately *adv.* 交替地,轮流地

ankle *n.* 踝关节,踝

bedpan *n.* (卧床病人用的)便盆

beneath *prep.* 在(或往)……下面(方)

bone *n.* 骨,骨头

chest *n.* 胸部,胸膛

complication *n.* 并发症

interval *n.* (时间上的)间隔,间歇

at regular intervals 每隔……时间,间或,不时

lateral *adj.* 侧面的,横向的

lateral position 侧卧位

lower back 腰背部

opposite *adj.* 对面的,另一边的; *n.* 对立面,反面

stress *n.* 压力,紧张,精神压力

undue *adj.* 过度的,不适当的

# SKILL 9
# Mouth Care

For the patient who is weak, unconscious, over-dry in the mouth or has dental ulcers, they easily get oral inflammations and infections. It is necessary to clean the oral mucosa and lingual surface in addition to the teeth. Special care may be needed every 2 to 8 hours according to the patient's oral health.

二维码 9-1

## PURPOSES

1. To keep the oral mucosa, the mouth and lips clean and moist.

2. To prevent halitosis and oral infections.

3. To improve appetite.

4. To keep the mouth healthy.

## ASSESSMENT

1. Assess the patient's condition, consciousness and ability of cooperation.

2. Identify presence of halitosis, inflammations and dentures.

3. Assess the oral mucosa to choose the proper mouthwash.

## PLANNING

### Equipment

1. Spatula

2. Foam swabs

3. Kidney dish

# 技能操作 9
# 口腔护理

虚弱、昏迷、口腔过度干燥或溃疡的病人易患口腔炎症和感染。护士应帮助病人清洗牙齿、口腔黏膜和舌面,或根据病人口腔健康状况,每 2～8 小时进行一次特殊口腔护理。

二维码 9-2

## 目的

1. 保持口腔黏膜及口唇清洁、湿润。

2. 预防口臭、口腔感染。

3. 促进食欲。

4. 保持口腔健康。

## 评估

1. 病情、意识状况及合作程度。

2. 是否有口臭、口腔炎症及有无假牙。

3. 口腔黏膜情况,选择合适的漱口溶液。

## 计划

### 用物准备

1. 压舌板

2. 海绵棒

3. 弯盘

4. Disposable protective pad or towel

5. Swabs

6. Mouthwash( e. g. , normal saline)

7. Flashlight

8. Clean gloves

9. Warm water

10. Drinking straw

11. Lip balm

12. Facial tissues

13. Mouth opener if needed

## IMPLEMENTATION

### Procedure

1. Clean natural teeth for a conscious but dependent patient：

(1) Perform hand hygiene and put on a mask.

(2) Carry the equipment to the bedside. Prior to performing the procedure, introduce yourself and verify the patient's identity. Explain the purposes of the procedure to the patient and tell him/her how to participate.

(3) Protect the patient's privacy by drawing the curtains around the bed or closing the door of the room.

(4) Assist the patient to turn his/her head to the nurse.

(5) Place a towel or a protective pad under the patient's chin and place the kidney dish against the patient's chin and lower cheek in order to collect the fluid from the mouth later.

(6) Put on clean gloves.

1) Moisten the patient's lips with wet swabs and ask the patient to sip warm water with a drinking straw to rinse the mouth. Inspect the oral cavity with the aid of a flashlight and a spatula. Examine the mouth condition involving moisture, cleanliness, presence of infected or bleeding areas, ulcers, etc.

2) Use a foam swab moistened with mouthwash to wipe all outer and inner surfaces of the teeth with an up-and-down motion. Clean the biting surface by placing the swab over the molars and moving it back and forth, like brushing the teeth. Then, carefully and gently,

4.一次性护理垫或毛巾

5.棉签

6.漱口溶液(如生理盐水)

7.手电筒

8.清洁手套

9.温水

10.吸水管

11.润唇膏

12.面巾纸

13.必要时备张口器

## 实施

### 操作步骤

1.为生活不能自理的清醒病人清洗牙齿:

(1)洗手,戴口罩。

(2)携用物至床旁,操作前自我介绍,确认病人。向病人解释操作内容、目的和配合方法。

(3)拉上床边围帘或关门以保护病人隐私。

(4)协助病人头偏向护士侧。

(5)铺毛巾或护理垫于颌下,置弯盘于口角旁接取漱口水。

(6)戴清洁手套。

1)用湿棉签湿润口唇,嘱病人用吸管吸温水漱口,用手电筒和压舌板检查口腔情况,包括口腔湿润度、清洁度,有无炎症、出血及溃疡等。

2)用海绵棒蘸取漱口溶液,似刷牙状纵向擦洗牙齿内、外面,由内向外来回擦洗咬合面。动作轻柔、仔细地按顺序擦洗两侧面颊、腭、舌面及舌下。

clean all the other tissues in the given order: the inside of the cheeks, the palate and the tongue.

3) Provide the patient with warm water or mouthwash. Ask the patient to rinse the mouth thoroughly and then spit it into the dish.

4) Make the patient repeat rinsing until the mouth is clean.

2. Clean natural teeth for an unconscious patient:

(1) Assist the patient to a lateral position with the head of the bed lowered. **Rationale**: *In this position, the mouthwash automatically runs out by gravity rather than being aspirated into the lungs.* If the patient's head cannot be lowered, turn it to one side. **Rationale**: *The fluid will readily run out of the mouth or pool in one side of the mouth, where it can be suctioned.*

(2) Remove the pillow and keep the mouth open with a mouth opener, leaving it between the molars.

(3) Clean the teeth and mouth by following the procedures previously described for a conscious patient.

(4) Rinse the patient's mouth by drawing about 10 mL of warm water or mouthwash into the syringe and injecting it gently into each side of the mouth. **Rationale**: *If the liquid is injected with force, some of it may flow down the patient's throat and be aspirated into the lungs.*

(5) Check carefully to make sure that all mouthwash has streamed from the mouth. If not, use the syringe to suck the fluid from the mouth. **Rationale**: *Fluids remaining in the mouth may be aspirated into the lungs.*

(6) Repeat flushing the oral cavity until the mouth is clean.

3. Dry around the patient's mouth with facial tissues, and remove the kidney dish and the protective pad.

4. Inspect the oral cavity with the aid of a flashlight and a spatula again.

5. Deal with the abnormal oral mucosa with appropriate medicine. Lubricate the patient's lips with a lip balm. **Rationale**: *Prevent cracking and subsequent infections.*

3）提供温水或漱口溶液，嘱病人用力漱口，将漱口溶液吐至弯盘。

4）重复漱口至口腔清洁。

2.为意识不清病人清洗牙齿：

（1）协助病人侧卧，摇低床头。**依据**：此体位借重力作用使漱口溶液从口腔中流出，避免误吸。如病情不允许摇低床头，则将病人头侧向一边。**依据**：头侧向一边使漱口溶液易于流出，或可积聚于一侧面颊部，便于抽吸。

（2）移去枕头。在臼齿间放置张口器助其张口。

（3）清洗牙齿及口腔，方法同清醒病人。

（4）用注射器抽取约 10 mL 温水或漱口溶液轻轻注入两侧面颊部进行冲洗。**依据**：用力过度可致误吸。

（5）仔细查看口腔，确认全部漱口溶液已流出，必要时用注射器抽出。**依据**：残留溶液可致误吸。

（6）重复冲洗至口腔清洁。

3.用面巾纸擦干口周，撤去弯盘和护理垫。

4.用手电筒及压舌板再次查看口腔情况。

5.用适当的药物处理口腔黏膜异常情况，涂润唇膏。**依据**：防止嘴唇裂开及感染。

6. Assist the patient to lie in a comfortable position.

7. Dispose of equipment appropriately.

8. Take off and discard the gloves.

9. Perform hand hygiene.

10. Document condition of the teeth, tongue, gums and oral mucosa, noting any problem such as ulcers and inflammations of the oral cavity, bleeding and swelling of the gums.

## EVALUATION

1. Report any abnormal findings to the doctor.

2. Implement necessary nursing interventions according to the patient's oral condition.

3. Conduct an ongoing assessment of the oral cavity or refer the patient to the dentist if necessary.

6. 协助病人取舒适体位。

7. 合理处置用物。

8. 脱下手套，弃置。

9. 洗手。

10. 记录牙齿、舌头、牙龈及口腔黏膜情况，如口腔溃疡、炎症，牙龈出血、肿胀等。

## 评价

1. 如口腔有异常情况，报告医生。

2. 根据病人口腔情况实施必要的护理。

3. 必要时进行口腔的后续评估或转诊牙医。

## Words and Expressions

appetite n. 食欲，胃口

aspirate vt. 吸入

cavity n. 腔，洞，孔

cheek n. 面颊，脸颊

chin n. 下巴，颏

cracking n. 裂缝，裂痕

dentist n. 牙科医生

denture n. 假牙

gravity n. 重力

gum n. 牙龈，齿龈，牙床

halitosis n. 口臭

inflammation n. 发炎，炎症

inject vt. (给……)注射(药物等)

injection n. 注射

lubricate vt. 给……上润滑油，上油

moisten vt. (使)变得潮湿，变得润滑

molar n. 臼齿；磨牙

mouthwash n. 漱口溶液，漱口剂

mucosa n. 黏膜

oral adj. 口头的

oral cavity 口腔

palate n. 腭

refer v. 把……送交给(以求获得帮助等)；参考，谈及

straw n. 吸管；稻草，麦秆

subsequent adj. 后来的，随后的

syringe n. 注射器

ulcer n. 溃疡

# SKILL 10
# Assessing Vital Signs

The traditional vital signs are body temperature, pulse, respiratory rate and blood pressure, often notated as 'T, P, R, BP'. Vital signs are taken to help assess the status of the body's vital functions. Taking a patient's vital signs should not be an automatic or routine procedure; it should be a thoughtful and scientific assessment. When and how often to take a patient's vital signs is chiefly nursing judgement, depending on the patient's health status.

二维码 10-1

## 10-1　Assessing Body Temperature

### PURPOSES

1. To identify if the body temperature is within the normal range.
2. To identify changes in body temperature after administering special medications (e. g. , antipyretic, immunosuppressants)

### ASSESSMENT

1. Assess clinical signs of hyperthermia or hypothermia.
2. Check the most appropriate body site for measurement.
3. Check condition of the measuring site.
4. Assess the patient's ability of cooperation.
5. Assess factors that may change body temperature.

# 技能操作 10
# 生命体征测量法

传统生命体征包括体温、脉搏、呼吸和血压,通常以"T、P、R、BP"来表示。测量生命体征有助于评估机体脏器的主要功能。测量生命体征不应是一项机械或例行操作,而应是全面、科学的评估。护士应根据病人的健康状况,确定测量生命体征的时间和次数。

二维码 10-2

## 10-1　体温测量法

### 目的

1.判断体温是否在正常范围内。
2.判断使用特殊药物(如退热剂、免疫抑制剂等)后体温的变化。

### 评估

1.体温过高或过低的临床体征。
2.最佳测温部位。

3.测温部位情况。
4.合作程度。
5.影响体温的因素。

## PLANNING

### Equipment

1. Thermometer

(1) Mercury thermometer (oral, rectal) (see Figure 10-1)

(2) Electronic/digital thermometer (see Figure 10-2)

(3) Infrared tympanic thermometer (see Figure 10-3)

(4) Non-contact infrared forehead temperature gun (see Figure 10-4)

2. Thermometer sheath or cover (for an electronic thermometer or a tympanic thermometer)

3. Liquid paraffin (for rectal temperature)

4. Clean gloves (for rectal temperature)

5. Paper tissues

## 计划

### 用物准备

1. 体温计

（1）水银体温计（口表、肛表）（见图 10-1）

（2）电子体温计（见图 10-2）

（3）红外线耳式体温计（见图 10-3）

（4）非接触红外线额式体温计（见图 10-4）

2. 体温计保护套（用电子体温计或耳温计时）

3. 液体石蜡（测肛温时）

4. 清洁手套（测肛温时）

5. 纸巾

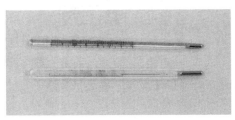

Figure 10-1　Mercury thermometers：*upper*—rectal，*lower*—oral

图 10-1　水银体温计：上—肛表，下—口表

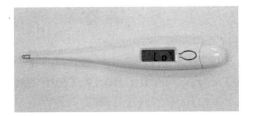

Figure 10-2　An electronic thermometer

图 10-2　电子体温计

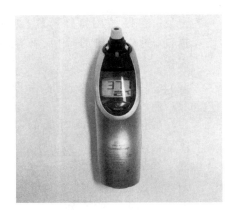

Figure 10-3　An infrared tympanic thermometer

图 10-3　红外线耳式体温计

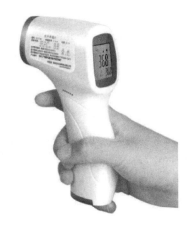

Figure 10-4　A non-contact infrared forehead temperature gun

图 10-4　非接触红外线额式体温计

## IMPLEMENTATION

### Preparation

1. Ensure that all equipment is functioning normally and the thermometer has been recently calibrated and maintained (otherwise it may cause erroneous measurement results).

2. Rinse the mercury thermometer with cold water after being disinfected with a chemical solution. Wipe it dry with a paper tissue or gauze.

3. For the mercury thermometer, ensure that the reading is below 35℃. If not, hold it at the glass end and shake it down, far from any object.

4. For the digital thermometer, simply press the button to turn it on.

### Procedure

1. Perform hand hygiene.

2. Identify the patient.

3. Explain the procedure to the patient and promote cooperation.

4. Protect the patient's privacy.

5. Place the patient in an appropriate position (e. g., the lateral position for inserting a rectal thermometer).

6. Place the thermometer.

(1) Mercury thermometer:

—Oral: Place the bulb tip on either side of the frenulum, underneath the tongue (see Figure 10-5). Instruct the patient to close the mouth but not the teeth.

## 实施

### 准备

1.确定用物性能良好,体温计已校准和维护(否则可致测量结果错误)。

2.经化学消毒液浸泡的水银体温计在使用前应用冷水冲净,然后用纸巾或纱布擦干。

3.确定水银体温计读数在35℃以下,否则手握体温计玻璃端将其甩下,勿触及其他物品。

4.电子体温计只需按下启动按钮。

### 操作步骤

1.洗手。

2.确认病人。

3.做好解释并取得配合。

4.保护病人隐私。

5.帮助病人取合适体位(如测肛温时取侧卧位)。

6.放置体温计。

(1)水银体温计:

——测口温:将体温计汞端放于病人左或右侧舌系带旁(见图 10-5),嘱病人紧闭口唇,勿咬。

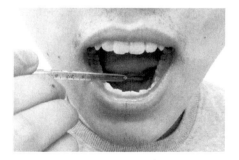

Figure 10-5　Placing an oral thermometer

图 10-5　口表放置

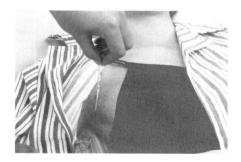

Figure 10-6　Placing the tip of the thermometer in the center of the axilla

图 10-6　体温计汞端放于腋窝正中

—Rectal：Put on clean gloves. Lubricate the bulb. Instruct the patient to take a slow deep breath during insertion. Never force the thermometer if resistance is felt. Insert for 3 to 4 cm in adults，2.5 cm in a child and 1.5 cm in an infant. Provide assistance if needed.

—Axillary：Wipe the axilla dry with paper tissues (if it's very moist). Place the thermometer at the center of the armpit (see Figure 10-6) and ask the patient to flex the same arm and place it over the chest to keep the thermometer in place.

(2) Tympanic thermometer：Straighten the ear canal，pull the pinna slightly upward and backward for adults. For children，gently pull it straight back. Apply a probe cover. Point the probe towards the eardrum. Using circular motion，slowly insert the probe until it fits into the ear canal. Press the button until the beep sound is heard.

(3) Electronic thermometer：Apply a thermometer sheath and take temperature the same as for a mercury thermometer.

7. Wait the appropriate amount of time.

(1) Mercury thermometer：3 min for oral and rectal temperature. 5-10 min for axillary temperature.

(2) Electronic and tympanic thermometers will indicate that the reading is complete with a light or a tone.

8. Remove the thermometer and discard the cover.

9. Wipe with a paper tissue if necessary. If gloves were put on，remove and discard them.

10. Read the temperature.

—The mercury thermometer：Hold the stem horizontally at the eye level. Locate the mercury line and check the temperature.

—The electronic and tympanic thermometers：Simply read the number displayed on the screen.

If the temperature is obviously too high, too low or inconsistent with the patient's condition, retake it with another thermometer which is working properly.

——测肛温：护士戴清洁手套，润滑肛表汞端。嘱病人做深慢呼吸，插入肛表时如遇阻力勿强行插入。成人插入 3～4 cm，儿童插入 2.5 cm，婴儿插入 1.5 cm。必要时协助测温。

——测腋温：用纸巾擦干腋窝(如潮湿)，将体温计汞端放于腋窝正中紧贴皮肤(见图 10-6)，嘱病人屈臂过胸夹紧体温计。

(2)耳式体温计：成人将耳郭向上向后、小儿向后轻轻拉直耳道。耳温计探头套上保护套，旋转探头，缓慢向鼓膜方向伸入使之与耳道贴合。按下测温键，听到蜂鸣声提示测量完毕。

(3)电子体温计：套上体温计保护套，测量方法同水银体温计。

7. 等待合适的测温时间。

(1)水银体温计：口温及肛温测 3 分钟，腋温测 5～10 分钟。

(2)电子体温计及耳式体温计测温完毕有亮光或声音提示。

8. 取出体温计，弃去保护套。

9. 需要时用纸巾擦拭体温计，如戴手套则脱去手套。

10. 读取体温值。

——水银体温计：持体温计与视线平，水银线所指刻度即为体温值。

——电子体温计及耳式体温计：读取显示屏上数值。

如体温值明显偏高、偏低或与病人病情不符，取另一性能良好的体温计重新测量。

11. Perform hand hygiene.

12. Wash and sterilize the thermometer if necessary.

13. Document the temperature in the patient's record.

**EVALUATION**

• Analyze the abnormal temperature reading considering other vital signs and influencing factors, and conduct appropriate nursing interventions such as adjusting the room temperature, removing heavy coverings or administering medications as ordered.

11. 洗手。

12. 需要时清洗、消毒体温计。

13. 在病情记录单上记录。

**评价**

• 结合其他生命体征和影响因素分析异常体温,实施合适的护理,如调节室温、减少盖被或遵医嘱给药。

# Words and Expressions

administer *vt.* 给予,施用(药物)等

administration *n.* (药物的)施用,执行

antipyretic *n.* 退热剂

axilla/armpit/underarm *n.* 腋窝,腋下

axillary *adj.* 腋窝的,腋下的

blood pressure 血压

bulb *n.* 鳞茎状物(如体温计的球部);电灯泡

calibrate *vt.* 校准(刻度,以使测量准确)

erroneous *adj.* 错误的

forehead *n.* 额,前额

frenulum *n.* 系带

hyperthermia *n.* 体温过高,高热
　　(前缀 hyper- 表示"过度,过多")

hypothermia *n.* 体温过低,低体温
　　(前缀 hypo- 表示"在……下,低于,次于")

immunosuppressant *n.* 免疫抑制剂
　　(前缀 immuno- 表示"免疫")

inconsistent *adj.* 不一致的,相矛盾的

infrared *adj.* 红外线的

mercury *n.* 水银,汞

notate *vt.* 以符号表示

paraffin *n.* 石蜡

pinna *n.* 耳郭

rectal *adj.* 直肠的

rectum *n.* 直肠

sheath *n.* (工具的)套,护套

temperature *n.* 温度,体温,气温

thermometer *n.* 温度计,体温计
　　(前缀 therm-/thermo- 表示"热,热的")

tympanic *adj.* 鼓膜的,耳膜的

vital signs 生命体征

# 10-2   Assessing Peripheral Pulse

**PURPOSES**

1. To identify whether the pulse is normal.

2. To compare the pulse on both sides of the body.

3. To assess the patient's cardiac function indirectly.

# 10-2　脉搏测量法

**目的**

1. 判断脉搏有无异常。

2. 比较两侧肢体脉搏是否一致。

3. 间接评估心脏功能。

## ASSESSMENT

1. Assess clinical signs（e. g. ，dyspnea，pallor，cyanosis，palpitation）of cardiovascular alteration，other than pulse rate，rhythm or intensity.

2. Identify factors that may alter heart rate（e. g. ，activity level and emotional status）.

3. Check the most appropriate site for assessment.

## PLANNING

### Equipment

• Watch with a sweep-second hand or digital second indicator

## IMPLEMENTATION

### Preparation

• Choose a suitable time to take the patient's pulse. A patient who has been exercising needs to rest for 20 to 30 minutes to permit the increased heart beat to return to normal.

### Procedure

1. Perform hand hygiene.

2. Explain the procedure to the patient and promote cooperation.

3. Select a monitoring site. Generally we choose the radial pulse.

4. Assist the patient to a comfortable position. For a lying patient，the patient's arms can rest alongside the body with the palm facing down or inward. For a sitting patient，put his/her forearms on the thighs，with the palm facing down or inward.

5. Palpate the artery and count the pulse：

（1）Lightly place two or three middle fingertips on the pulse point（see Figure 10-7（a），（b））. **Rationale**：*Using the thumb is contraindicated because the thumb has a pulse of its own that the nurse may mistake for the patient's pulse.*

## 评估

1. 除脉率、脉律及脉搏强度外的其他心血管系统功能改变的临床体征（如呼吸困难、面色苍白、发绀、心悸）。

2. 影响心率的因素（如活动、情绪状态）。

3. 最佳测脉部位。

## 计划

### 用物准备

• 有秒针的手表或数字秒表

## 实施

### 准备

• 选择合适的测脉时间。测脉前若有运动，应休息20～30分钟，使心率平复后再测量。

### 操作步骤

1. 洗手。

2. 向病人解释并取得配合。

3. 选择测量部位，临床上最常使用桡动脉。

4. 协助病人取舒适体位。病人取半卧位时，嘱病人手臂放于身体两侧，掌心向下或向内；取坐位时将手放在大腿上，掌心向下或向内。

5. 测量脉搏：

（1）中间两个或三个手指尖轻轻放于脉搏搏动点上方（见图10-7（a），（b））。**依据**：勿用拇指诊脉，因自己的拇指小动脉搏动易与病人的脉搏相混淆。

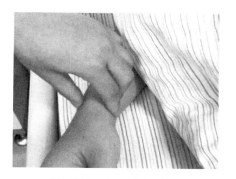 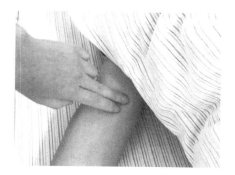

(a) Taking the radial pulse
(a) 测量桡动脉脉搏

(b) Taking the brachial pulse
(b) 测量肱动脉脉搏

Figure 10-7   Taking the pulse

图 10-7   测脉搏

（2）Count the beats for 30 seconds and multiply the result by 2. If you're taking a patient's pulse for the first time (when obtaining baseline data), or if the patient is critically ill, presents abnormal pulse, or is a baby, count for a full minute. **Rationale**: *A 1-minute count provides a more accurate assessment of an irregular pulse than a 30-second count*. If an abnormal pulse is found, it is required to take the heart rate as well.

6. Assess the pulse rhythm and intensity:

（1）Assess the pulse rhythm by noting pulse intervals. Normal pulse has equal intervals.

（2）Assess the pulse intensity. Normal pulse can be felt with moderate pressure, and the intensity of each beat is equal.

（3）If pulse deficit occurs, two nurses are needed to take the pulse at the same time. One takes the pulse rate, and the other listens to the heart beat with the stethoscope. The nurse with the stethoscope gives the instructions to start and stop. Count for 1 minute.

7. Document the pulse rate, rhythm, intensity and your actions in the patient's record.

## EVALUATION

• Analyze the abnormal pulse in combination with other vital signs and influencing factors. Conduct appropriate nursing interventions such as administering medications as ordered.

（2）计数 30 秒乘以 2。如为首次测脉（获取基础资料）或为危重、脉搏异常及婴幼儿测脉应计数 1 分钟。**依据**：1 分钟比 30 秒更能准确地测出异常脉搏。脉搏异常者还需测心率。

6. 评估脉律及强度：

（1）以脉搏的间隔时间评估脉律，正常脉搏跳动间隔时间相等。

（2）评估脉搏强度，正常脉搏以中等的指压力量即可测得，每搏强弱相等。

（3）如出现脉搏短绌，需由两名护士同时测量，一人测脉率，一人使用听诊器测心率。由测心率者发出开始和停止的指令，计数 1 分钟。

7. 在病情记录单上记录脉率、脉律、脉搏强度及实施的护理。

## 评价

• 结合其他生命体征和影响因素分析异常脉搏，实施合适的护理，如遵医嘱给药等。

# Words and Expressions

alongside *prep*. 在……旁边,沿着……边

alter *vt*. 改变,更改,改动

alteration *n*. 改变,变化

arterial *adj*. 动脉的

   (前缀 arteri-/arterio- 表示"动脉")

artery *n*. 动脉

beat *n*.(心脏等的)跳动;*vt*. 打,打败

cardiac *adj*. 心脏的

cardiovascular *adj*. 心血管的

   (前缀 cardi-/cardio- 表示"心,心脏")

critically *adv*. 可能有危险地,严重地

cyanosis *n*.(医学)发绀,青紫

deficit *n*. 缺少,亏损

dyspnea *n*. 呼吸困难

   (前缀 dys- 表示"困难的,不良的";后缀 -pnea表示"呼吸")

intensity *n*. 强度,强烈

irregular *adj*. 不规则的,无规律的

multiply *v*. 乘,乘以

pallor *n*. 苍白(尤指脸色)

palpate *vt*. 触诊,触摸检查

palpitation *n*. 心悸

peripheral *adj*. 外围的,周边的

   (前缀 peri- 表示"周围,邻近")

radial *adj*. 桡骨的

rhythm *n*. 节奏,律动

sweep *n*. 摆动;*vt*. 清扫

## 10-3　Assessing Respiration

### PURPOSES

1. To identify abnormal respiration and its pattern.

2. To monitor respiration after administering anesthetic or other medications which may influence respiration.

### ASSESSMENT

1. Assess skin and mucous membrane color (e. g. , cyanosis, pallor).

2. Assess the patient's position.

3. Assess dyspnea.

4. Identify medications affecting respiration.

### PLANNING

#### Equipment

• Watch with a sweep second hand or digital second indicator

## 10-3　呼吸测量法

### 目的

1.识别异常呼吸及其形态。

2.观察使用麻醉药或其他影响呼吸的药物后病人的呼吸情况。

### 评估

1.皮肤及黏膜颜色(如发绀、苍白)。

2.病人体位。

3.呼吸困难情况。

4.影响呼吸的药物。

### 计划

#### 用物准备

• 有秒针的手表或数字秒表

# IMPLEMENTATION

## Preparation

• For a routine measurement of respiration, choose a suitable time. A patient who has been exercising needs to rest for 20 to 30 minutes to permit the increased respiratory rate to return to normal.

## Procedure

1. Perform hand hygiene.

2. Explain to the patient what you are going to do, why it is necessary and how he/she can cooperate to lessen the patient's anxiety and promote cooperation.

3. Observe and count the respiratory rate:

(1) Once the patient realizes that you are taking his/her respiration, he/she will change the respiration pattern voluntarily. In order to prevent this, pretend to take the radial pulse while observing the chest or abdomen movement for the count of breathing.

(2) Count breath for 30 seconds and multiply the number by 2. Infants and patients with abnormal respiration require a full minute. Repeat if necessary. An exhalation plus an inhalation counts as once.

4. Observe the depth, rhythm and character of respiration.

(1) Observe the depth of respiration by watching the movement of the chest or abdomen. **Rationale**: *During deep respiration, a large volume of air is exchanged; during shallow respiration, a small volume is exchanged.*

(2) Observe if the respiration has regular or irregular rhythm. **Rationale**: *Normal respiration has equal intervals.*

(3) If the patient's breathing is weak, place little cotton fiber near the patient's nostril to count respiration.

(4) Observe the character of respiration: the sound produced and the effort required. **Rationale**: *Normal, respiration is silent and effortless.*

# 实施

## 准备

• 选择适宜的时间进行常规呼吸测量。测量前如有活动,应休息20～30分钟,使呼吸平复后再测量。

## 操作步骤

1. 洗手。

2. 向病人解释操作内容、目的和方法,以减轻病人焦虑并取得配合。

3. 观察、测量呼吸:

(1)病人意识到自己被测呼吸时会有意识地改变呼吸形态。护士应将手放在诊脉部位似诊脉状,同时观察病人胸部或腹部的起伏。

(2)如呼吸无异常,计数30秒乘以2;呼吸异常者和婴儿须计数1分钟;必要时重测。一呼一吸为1次。

4. 观察呼吸的深度、节律和特征。

(1)观察病人胸腹起伏以判断呼吸深浅。**依据**:深呼吸时潮气量大,浅表呼吸时潮气量小。

(2)观察呼吸节律是否规则。**依据**:正常呼吸间隔时间相等。

(3)呼吸微弱病人可置少许棉花纤维于鼻孔前,观察棉花纤维吹动的次数。

(4)观察呼吸特征:呼吸声音、呼吸是否费力。**依据**:正常呼吸无声且不费力。

5. Document the respiratory rate, depth, rhythm and character in the patient's record.

5.记录呼吸频率、深度、节律及特征。

## EVALUATION

1. Analyze the abnormal respiration and respiratory pattern in association with other vital signs and influencing factors.

2. Conduct appropriate nursing interventions such as repositioning the patient to breathe easily, administering oxygen or appropriate medications as ordered.

## 评价

1.结合其他生命体征和影响因素分析异常呼吸及其形态。

2.实施合适的护理,如协助病人取利于呼吸的体位、吸氧或遵医嘱给药。

## Words and Expressions

effortless *adj.* 容易的,不费力气的
　(后缀-less 表示"没有……的,不,无")
exhalation *n.* 呼气,呼出
exhale *v.* 呼气,吐出(肺中的空气、烟等)
inhalation *n.* 吸入

inhale *vt.* 吸入,吸气
lessen *vt.* (使)变小,减轻,变少
nostril *n.* 鼻孔
respiration *n.* 呼吸
voluntarily *adv.* 自愿地,主动地

# 10-4　Assessing Blood Pressure

## PURPOSES

1. To identify and monitor changes in blood pressure.

2. To identify presence or history of cardiovascular diseases indirectly.

## ASSESSMENT

1. Check symptoms and signs of hypertension (e. g., headache, blurred vision, chest distress, palpitation, vomiting).

2. Check symptoms and signs of hypotension (e. g., dizziness, syncope, shock).

3. Check factors affecting blood pressure (e. g., activity, emotional stress, pain, and time the patient last smoked or ingested caffeine).

# 10-4　血压测量法

## 目的

1.判断和监测异常血压。

2.间接判断是否有心血管系统疾病或病史。

## 评估

1.高血压的症状和体征(如头痛、视物模糊、胸闷、心悸、呕吐)。

2.低血压的症状和体征(如头昏、晕厥、休克)。

3.影响血压的因素(如运动、情绪紧张、疼痛、病人最后一次吸烟或摄入咖啡因的时间)。

# PLANNING

## Equipment

1. Mercury sphygmomanometer（with a pressure cuff of the appropriate size）（see Figures 10-8, 10-9）, aneroid sphygmomanometer（see Figure 10-10）or electronic sphygmomanometer（see Figure 10-11）

2. Stethoscope（see Figures 10-12, 10-13）

# 计划

## 用物准备

1. 水银血压计（袖带宽窄适宜）（见图 10-8、图 10-9）、无液血压计（见图 10-10）或电子血压计（见图 10-11）

2. 听诊器（见图 10-12、图 10-13）

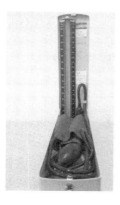

Figure 10-8　A mercury manometer
图 10-8　水银血压计

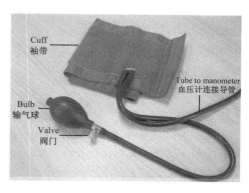

Figure 10-9　A blood pressure cuff
图 10-9　血压计袖带

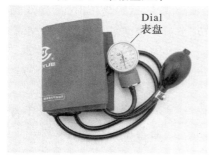

Figure 10-10　An aneroid manometer with a dial
图 10-10　无液血压计及表盘

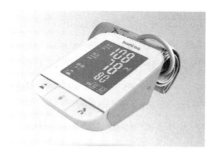

Figure 10-11　An electronic manometer
图 10-11　电子血压计

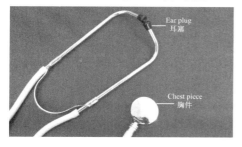

Figure 10-12　A stethoscope
图 10-12　听诊器

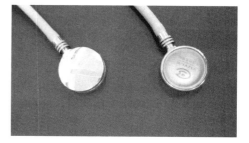

Figure 10-13　Two sides of a chest piece: Drum（left）and diaphragm（right）
图 10-13　听诊器胸件两面:鼓面（左）及膜面（右）

# IMPLEMENTATION

## Preparation

1. Ensure that the equipment is intact and functioning properly. Check the rubber tubing for air leak.

2. Make sure that the patient was not smoking, ingesting caffeine, exercising, and was not agitated or in pain, within 30 minutes before measurement. **Rationale**: *These can result in a temporary increase in the blood pressure.*

## Procedure

1. Perform hand hygiene.

2. Explain to the patient what you are going to do, why it is necessary and how he/she can cooperate to lessen the patient's anxiety and promote cooperation.

3. Protect the patient's privacy.

4. Position the patient appropriately:

(1) An adult patient could be either in a sitting or a lying position.

(2) In a sitting position, the patient's both feet should be flat on the floor. **Rationale**: *Legs crossed at the knee results in elevated systolic and diastolic blood pressure.* The elbow should be slightly bended with the palm facing up and the forearm supported at heart level.

(3) In a lying position, the patient's arm naturally extends alongside the midaxillary line, with the palm facing up.

(4) Apart from the forearm, readings in any other position should be specified. The blood pressure is normally similar in sitting, standing and lying positions, but it can vary significantly if the patients is not positioned properly. **Rationale**: *The reading increases when the arm is below the heart level and decreases when the arm is above the heart level.*

(5) Expose the upper arm and remove tight or restrictive clothing.

5. Locate the brachial artery (see Figure 10-7 (b)). Wrap the deflated cuff evenly around the upper

# 实施

## 准备

1. 用物齐全,性能良好,血压计橡胶管无漏气。

2. 确定病人在测量前 30 分钟无吸烟、摄入咖啡因、运动、情绪激动及疼痛。依据:此类因素可使血压暂时升高。

## 操作步骤

1. 洗手。

2. 向病人解释操作内容、目的和方法,以减轻病人焦虑并取得配合。

3. 保护病人隐私。

4. 协助病人取合适的体位:

(1)成年病人可取坐位或仰卧位。

(2)坐位时,病人双脚应平放于地面。依据:两腿交叉可使收缩压和舒张压升高。肘微屈,掌心向上,手臂与心脏平齐。

(3)仰卧时,病人手臂自然伸直与腋中线平齐,掌心向上。

(4)除上臂血压外,应注明测量部位。坐位、站立位及仰卧位测得的血压值一般无差异。如体位不当可使测得的血压有较大差异。依据:手臂高于心脏水平可使测得的血压值偏低,而手臂低于心脏水平则使血压值偏高。

(5)露出上臂,宽松衣袖。

5. 触及肱动脉搏动(见图10-7(b))。驱尽袖带内空气,将袖

arm with the center of the bladder directly on the artery. **Rationale**：*The bladder inside the cuff must be placed directly on the artery to compress blood flow in order to get the accurate reading*. A finger's space under the cuff is the best (see Figure 10-14).

For an adult, place the lower border of the cuff approximately 2 to 3 cm above the antecubital space.

6. If this is the patient's initial examination, perform a preliminary palpation to determine the systolic pressure：

（1）Palpate the brachial (or radial) artery with the fingertips.

（2）Turn off the valve of the bulb.

（3）Pump the bladder until you no longer feel the pulse. Take note of the pressure on the manometer when the pulse disappears. **Rationale**：*This is to estimate the systolic pressure*.

（4）Deflate and wait for 1 to 2 minutes before taking another measurement. **Rationale**：*A waiting period gives the blood trapped in the veins time to be released. Otherwise, a false high systolic reading will occur*.

带的橡胶气囊中部正对肱动脉上方平整地缠于上臂中部。**依据**：为使血压测量准确，橡胶气囊应正对肱动脉上方以压迫血流。松紧以能放入一指为宜(见图 10-14)。

若病人为成人，血压计袖带下缘距肘窝 2~3 cm。

6.如病人为初次测量血压，实施初步触诊法确定病人收缩压。

（1）用手指触及肱动脉(或桡动脉)搏动。

（2）关闭输气球阀门。

（3）打气至肱动脉(或桡动脉)搏动消失，记下此时的血压值。**依据**：此法可估计收缩压。

（4）驱尽袖带内空气，1~2 分钟后重测。**依据**：间歇 1~2 分钟可使袖带下方滞留的静脉血液流散；否则可使测得的收缩压值偏高。

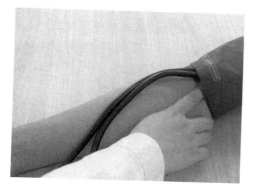

Figure 10-14　A finger's space under the cuff is the best

图 10-14　袖带松紧以能插入一指为宜

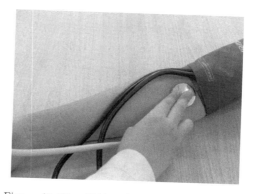

Figure 10-15　Taking brachial blood pressure. Note：How the stethoscope is held against the arm

图 10-15　测肱动脉血压时听诊器胸件的放置

7. Properly place the stethoscope：

（1）Insert the eartips of the stethoscope slightly forward in your ears. **Rationale**：*It sounds more clearly when the eartips are in the direction of the ear canal*.

（2）Place the diaphragm of the stethoscope directly on the brachial pulse site beside the cuff.

7.正确放置听诊器：

（1）耳塞朝前戴好听诊器。**依据**：听诊器耳塞顺耳道方向戴入使声音更清晰。

（2）将听诊器胸件的膜面紧贴皮肤放于肱动脉搏动最明显

**Rationale**：*This is to avoid noise made from rubbing the amplifier against cloth.*

（3）Hold the chestpiece with the fingers（see Figure 10-15），avoid inserting it under the cuff or clothing.

8. Take the patient's blood pressure：

（1）Pump up the bladder until the manometer reads 20 to 30 mmHg after the brachial pulse disappeared.

（2）Slowly release the cuff's valve so that the pressure decreases at the rate of 4 mmHg per second.

**Rationale**：*A faster rate results in a lower blood pressure reading than the actual blood pressure while a slower rate results in a higher reading.*

（3）As the pressure in the cuff falls，note the point at which the first sound is heard. It is the systolic blood pressure. The point at which the muffled sound disappears，is the diastolic blood pressure.

（4）Deflate the cuff rapidly and completely.

（5）Wait for 1 to 2 minutes before measuring again（if required）.

（6）Repeat the above steps once or twice to ensure accuracy or if the sound is unclear.

（7）If the two readings differ by more than 5 mmHg，additional measurement is required. Take the average of 3 results.

9. If this is the patient's initial examination，repeat the procedure on the patient's other arm. There should be a difference of no more than 10 mmHg between two arms. The arm with the higher pressure should be the one used for subsequent examinations.

**Variation：taking blood pressure by palpation**

If it is not possible to use a stethoscope to take blood pressure，or if the Korotkoff sounds cannot be heard，palpate the radial or brachial artery while the cuff is released. The manometer reading at the point where the pulse reappears stands for the systolic blood pressure.

**Variation：taking a thigh blood pressure**

（1）Help the patient to take a prone position. If the patient cannot take this position，measure blood

处。**依据**：避免听诊器胸件和衣服摩擦产生杂音。

（3）用手指轻按胸件（见图 10-15），不可塞入袖带下。

8.测量血压：

（1）打气至肱动脉搏动音消失后再使汞柱上升 20～30 mmHg。

（2）缓慢放气，速度以水银柱每秒下降 4 mmHg 为宜。**依据**：放气速度过快可使测得的血压值偏低，过慢则使血压值偏高。

（3）随着水银柱的下降，听到第一声搏动音时水银柱所指的刻度即为收缩压；当搏动音消失时水银柱所指的刻度即为舒张压。

（4）测量完毕，快速驱尽袖带内空气。

（5）如需重测，须间隔 1～2 分钟。

（6）为了保证测量准确性或当血压听不清时，应重复测量 1～2 次。

（7）如两次血压值差别在 5 mmHg 以上，应再次测量，取 3 次读数的平均值。

9.初诊者应测量另一侧肢体血压。两侧肢体的血压差应在 10 mmHg 以内，后续测量应选择血压高的一侧肢体。

**触诊法测量血压**

如不能用听诊器听诊血压或柯氏音听不清，可用手指触摸桡动脉或肱动脉的搏动，随着缓慢放气，摸到第一次搏动时水银柱所指刻度即为收缩压。

**下肢血压测量法**

（1）协助病人取俯卧位，如病人不能俯卧，可取仰卧位，膝部微

pressure when the patient is in a supine position with his/her knees slightly bended so that the stethoscope can be placed in the popliteal space.

（2）Expose the thigh, taking care not to expose the patient too long.

（3）Locate the popliteal artery. Wrap the deflated cuff evenly around the midthigh with the bladder in the popliteal space and the bottom edge of the cuff 3 to 5 cm above the popliteal space. **Rationale**：*The bladder must be directly on the popliteal artery to ensure the accuracy of reading.*

（4）In adults, the systolic pressure in the popliteal artery is usually 20 to 30 mmHg higher than that in the brachial artery because of the larger bladder. The diastolic pressure is usually the same.

**Variation：Using an electronic blood pressure monitor**

（1）Place the cuff on the extremity according to the manufacturer's guidelines.

（2）Turn on the switch.

（3）Note the digital result when blood pressure readings come out.

10．Remove the cuff.

11．Tidy up the sphygmomanometer. If a mercury manometer is used, tilt the cover of the manometer 45° to the right side to make the mercury flow back to the groove, then turn off the valve. Place the cuff in the case properly.

12．Assist the patient in returning to a comfortable position.

13．Document and report measuring data. Record two pressures in the form '120/80' in which '120' is the systolic pressure and '80' is the diastolic pressure. Record a difference greater than 10 mmHg between the two arms or legs.

## EVALUATION

1．Report any significant change in the patient's blood pressure.

屈以便将听诊器放于腘窝处。

（2）露出大腿，勿暴露过久。

（3）触及腘动脉，将血压计袖带平整地缠于大腿下部，使橡胶气囊对准腘窝正中，袖带下缘距腘窝3～5 cm。**依据**：为使测量结果准确，应将橡胶气囊正对腘动脉上方。

（4）因下肢血压计袖带的橡胶气囊较大，故成人下肢收缩压比上肢高20～30 mmHg，舒张压无差异。

**电子血压计测量法**
（1）按使用说明缠绕袖带。

（2）打开血压计开关开始测量血压。

（3）测量完毕，注意血压计显示屏上的血压值。

10．取下袖带。

11．整理血压计。如果是水银血压计，应将血压计盖子右倾45°，使水银全部流入汞槽内，关闭汞槽开关；整理袖带，放入盒内。

12．协助病人取舒适体位。

13．记录并报告测量结果。以"120/80"的形式记录血压值，120表示收缩压，80 为舒张压。如双上肢（或双下肢）之间的血压差在10 mmHg 以上，应做好记录。

## 评价

1．如病人血压有较大变化，应报告医生。

2. Conduct appropriate nursing interventions, such as administering medications as ordered. If the blood pressure is significantly higher or lower than usual，take appropriate safety precautions.

2.提供合适的护理,如遵医嘱给药。若血压明显高于或低于正常范围,应采取适当的安全防护措施。

## Words and Expressions

aneroid *adj*. 无液的;*n*. 无液气压计

antecubital *adj*. 肘前的

　　（前缀 ante- 表示"在……前,在……前面"）

bladder *n*. 皮囊;膀胱

blurred *adj*. 模糊不清的,难以区分的

brachial *adj*. 肱的,臂的

deflate *vt*. 放掉（轮胎、气球等的）气,使瘪下来

　　（前缀 de- 表示"……的反义,去掉,除掉"）

dial *n*. 刻度盘,表盘,控制盘

diastolic *adj*. 心脏舒张期的

diastolic blood pressure 舒张压

eartips/ear plugs *n*. 耳机,听筒

extremity *n*. （人体的）四肢,手足

groove *n*. 槽,沟,辙

hypertension *n*. 高血压

hypotension *n*. 低血压

ingest *vt*. 摄入,食入

Korotkoff sounds 柯氏音

manometer *n*. 测压计,血压计

manufacturer *n*. 生产商,制造者

midaxillary *adj*. 腋窝中间的

　　（前缀 mid- 表示"中,中部"）

midaxillary line 腋中线

muffled *adj*. 模糊不清的,沉闷的

popliteal *adj*. 腘的,腿后弯的

popliteal space 腘窝

preliminary *adj*. 初步的,开始的

prone *adj*. 俯卧的,易于遭受

prone position 俯卧位

pump *n*. 泵;*vt*. 用泵（或泵样器官等）输送

restrictive *adj*. 约束的,限制性的

significantly *adv*. 显著地,明显地,有重大意义地

supine *adj*. 仰卧的,平躺着的

supine position 仰卧位

symptom *n*. 症状,征兆

syncope *n*. 晕厥

systolic *adj*. 心脏收缩期的

systolic blood pressure 收缩压

temporary *adj*. 暂时的,临时的

valve *n*. 阀,阀门,气门

vomit *v*. 呕,吐;*n*. 呕吐物

# SKILL 11 Suctioning Secretions after Tracheostomy

# 技能操作 11 气管切开套管内吸痰法

The trachea and surrounding respiratory tissues are irritated after tracheostomy. Thus excessive secretions are produced. Suctioning is necessary to remove those secretions and maintain the airway unobstructed. The procedure is uncomfortable with potential risk of hypoxemia. Therefore, it should only be performed when indicated.

气管切开后,气管及其周围组织受套管刺激而产生过多分泌物。吸痰可清除套管内分泌物,保持气道通畅。吸痰可引起病人不适,还有潜在的缺氧危险,故应按需吸痰。

二维码 11-1

二维码 11-2

## PURPOSES

1. To maintain the airway patent.
2. To promote respiratory function.
3. To prevent pneumonia that results from accumulated secretions.

## ASSESSMENT

1. Assess the patient's condition, consciousness and mental status, ability of cooperation.

2. Assess cough reflex and the ability to remove the secretions through coughing.

3. Assess clinical signs indicating the need for suctioning: presence of secretions in the endotracheal tube, bubbling breath sounds when the chest is auscultated, high airway pressure or low tidal volume ventilation alarm, decreased oxygen saturation ($SaO_2$), tachypnea, etc.

## PLANNING

### Equipment

1. Sterile suction catheter of the appropriate size

## 目的

1. 保持病人气道通畅。
2. 促进呼吸功能。
3. 预防因痰液积聚而引起肺炎。

## 评估

1. 病情、意识和心理状态、合作程度。

2. 咳嗽反射及咳痰能力。

3. 吸痰指征:气管套管内有分泌物、肺部听诊可闻及痰鸣音、气道高压或低潮气量报警、氧饱和度下降、呼吸急促等。

## 计划

### 用物准备

1. 型号合适的无菌吸痰管

(see Figure 11-1)

　　2. Oxygen supply, flow meter

　　3. Portable suction machine or wall suction outlet (see Figure 11-2), wall suction regulator (see Figure 11-3), suction tubing, suction collection container

　　4. Resuscitation bag/Ambu bag (see Figure 11-4)

　　5. Stethoscope

　　6. Disposable sterile containers

　　7. Sterile solution (e. g., sterile normal saline, sterile water)

　　8. Sterile gloves

　　9. Sterile gauzes

　　10. Goggles or face shield (if needed)

　　11. Sputum trap (if needed)

（见图 11-1）

　　2. 氧气装备，氧气表

　　3. 便携式吸痰器或中心负压吸引出口（见图 11-2）、中心负压吸引表（见图 11-3）、橡胶导管、痰液收集瓶

　　4. 呼吸皮囊（见图 11-4）

　　5. 听诊器

　　6. 一次性无菌容器

　　7. 无菌溶液（如无菌生理盐水、无菌用水）

　　8. 无菌手套

　　9. 无菌纱布

　　10. 必要时备护目镜或防护面罩

　　11. 需收集痰标本时备集痰器

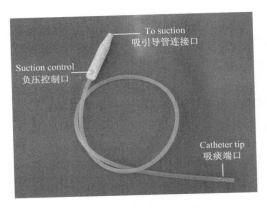

Figure 11-1　A suction catheter

图 11-1　吸痰管

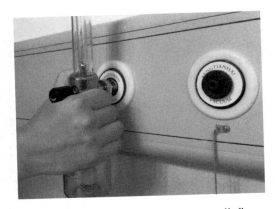

Figure 11-2　Inserting an oxygen wall flow meter into an axygen wall outlet (left). A suction wall outlet (right)

图 11-2　将氧气流量表插入中心供氧出口（左）；中心负压吸引出口（右）

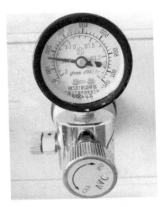

Figure 11-3　A wall suction regulator

图 11-3　中心负压吸引表

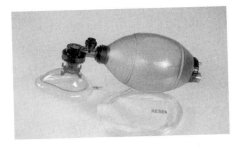

Figure 11-4　Resuscitation bag

图 11-4　呼吸皮囊

## IMPLEMENTATION

### Procedure

1. Perform hand hygiene and put on a mask.

2. Before performing the procedure, verify the patient's identity, and introduce yourself if the patient is conscious. Explain the procedure to the patient and ask for cooperation. Inform the patient that suctioning is uncomfortable, usually causes intermittent coughing, but it helps to remove the secretions and thus relieves breathing difficulty.

3. Protect the patient's privacy.

4. Prepare the patient:

(1) If not contraindicated, place the patient in the semi-Fowler's position to promote deep breathing, lung expansion and productive coughing. **Rationale**: *Deep breathing oxygenates the lungs, counteracts the hypoxic effects of suctioning, and may induce coughing, which helps to loosen and move secretions.*

(2) Dilute the patient's sputum by inhalating Budesonide nebulization with a tracheostomy mask, if needed.

(3) If the patient does not have copious secretions, hyperventilate the lungs with an resuscitation bag before suctioning:

1) Summon an assistant, if one is available.

2) Connect the resuscitator with 100% oxygen. If the patient is receiving oxygen, disconnect the oxygen source from the tracheostomy tube. Attach the Ambu bag to the tracheostomy tube.

3) Compress the Ambu bag 10 to 15 times as the patient inhales. This is best done by an assistant who can use both hands to compress the bag.

4) Observe the rise and fall of the patient's chest to assess the adequacy of tidal volume.

5) Remove the Ambu bag and place it on the patient's chest, with the connector facing up.

(4) If the patient has copious secretions, do not

## 实施

### 操作步骤

1.洗手,戴口罩。

2.操作前确认病人。如病人意识清醒,作自我介绍,向病人解释以取得配合。告知病人吸痰有不适感,会引起间歇性咳嗽,但咳嗽有助于清除痰液,改善呼吸困难。

3.保护病人隐私。

4.病人准备:

(1)如无禁忌,协助病人取半坐卧位以利深呼吸、肺扩张及有效咳嗽。**依据**:深呼吸使吸入氧量增加,可缓解吸痰引起的缺氧,并可诱发咳嗽,使痰液咳出。

(2)必要时在吸痰前通过气管切开面罩给予氧气雾化吸入布地奈德以稀释痰液。

(3)如病人痰液较少,吸痰前用呼吸皮囊鼓肺:

1)如有助手,请助手协助。

2)将呼吸皮囊连接纯氧,如病人正在吸氧,分离气管套管处氧气,将呼吸皮囊与气管套管相连。

3)病人吸气时,挤压呼吸皮囊10～15次。最好由助手用双手挤压皮囊。

4)观察病人胸部起伏情况以评估潮气量。

5)移开呼吸皮囊,放于病人胸前,连接口朝上。

(4)如病人痰液较多,不可用

hyperventilate with the Ambu bag. Instead：Adjust the oxygen flow to 8-10 L/min or the FiO₂ to 100% to hyperoxygenate the patient for 1 to 2 min before suctioning. **Rationale**：*Hyperventilating a patient who has copious secretions may force the secretions to flow deeper into the respiratory tract.*

5. Prepare the equipment for an open suction system：

(1) Turn the suction on and occlude the suction tubing to check if the equipment is working properly.

(2) Take out the sterile container (touching only the outside), and pour sterile solution or sterile water into the container.

(3) Open the suction catheter. Carefully expose the catheter connection in readiness for use.

(4) Put on a sterile glove for the dominant hand. Place its package paper on the patient's chest, below the tracheostomy.

(5) With the gloved hand, carefully take out the catheter from the package, hold the suction tubing in the non-dominant hand, and attach the suction catheter to the suction tubing.

(6) Turn on the suction and set the negative pressure. 100 to 120 mmHg is normally used for adults (maximum 200 mmHg).

6. Flush and lubricate the catheter：

(1) Using the gloved hand, put the catheter tip in the sterile solution.

(2) Using the thumb of the non-dominant hand, occlude the suction control port and suck a small amount of the sterile solution into the catheter. **Rationale**：*This aims to check if the suction equipment is working successfully and lubricate the outside and the inside of the catheter, which helps insert with less tissue trauma and prevents secretions from sticking to the inside of the catheter.*

7. Remove oxygen source and put it on the paper using your non-dominant hand.

8. Quickly and gently insert the catheter without applying suction：

呼吸皮囊鼓肺，而应在吸痰前将氧流量调至 8～10 L/min 或纯氧吸入 1～2 min。**依据**：痰液较多时鼓肺易使分泌物进入呼吸道深部。

5. 准备用物进行开放式吸痰：

(1)将橡胶导管折起，打开吸引器开关以检查吸引器性能。

(2)取出无菌容器（只能触及外面），倒入无菌溶液或无菌用水。

(3)打开吸痰管包装，小心露出吸痰管连接口备用。

(4)惯用手戴无菌手套，将手套包装纸放于病人胸前、气管切开口下方。

(5)用戴了手套的手小心取出吸痰管，另一手持橡胶导管，将其与吸痰管相连。

(6)打开吸引器开关，调节负压，成人一般 100～120 mmHg（不超过 200 mmHg）。

6. 冲洗、润滑吸痰管：

(1)惯用手持吸痰管，将其末端放入无菌溶液中。

(2)非惯用手的拇指按住负压控制口，吸引少量无菌溶液。**依据**：检查负压吸引器性能，同时润滑吸痰管内外面，以减少插管时对气管黏膜组织的损伤，防止痰液黏附在吸痰管内壁。

7. 用非惯用手移开氧气，放于胸前。

8. 在无负压状态下动作轻快地插入吸痰管：

(1) Release your thumb from the suction control port. Using your dominant hand, quickly and gently insert the catheter into the trachea through the tracheostomy tube. **Rationale**: *Suction is not applied during insertion in order to prevent tissue trauma and oxygen loss (see Figure 11-5).*

（1）松开控制口,惯用手持吸痰管轻快地将其插入套管内。**依据**:插管时不吸引以防气管黏膜损伤及氧气损耗(见图 11-5)。

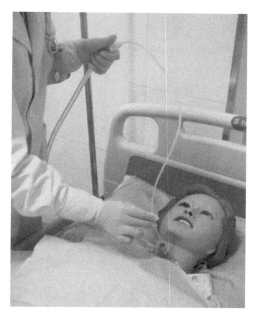

Figure 11-5  Inserting the catheter into the trachea through the tracheostomy tube. Note: Suction is not applied while inserting the catheter

图 11-5  将吸痰管从气管切开导管插入气管。注意:插管时不吸引

(2) Insert the catheter until the patient starts coughing or you feel resistance. Withdraw the catheter for about 1-2 cm before applying suction. **Rationale**: *Resistance usually means that the catheter tip has reached the bifurcation of the airway. Withdrawing the catheter prevents damaging the mucous membranes at the bifurcation.*

9. Perform suctioning:

(1) Occlude the control port with the non-dominant thumb and rotate the catheter with your dominant thumb and forefinger while slowly withdrawing it. **Rationale**: *Suctioning time is restricted to 8-10 seconds (no more than 15 s) to minimize oxygen loss.*

（2）插管至病人咳嗽或感到有阻力时将吸痰管上提 1～2 cm。**依据**:遇到阻力表示吸痰管已达气管分叉处,上提 1～2 cm 再开始吸引,以防止气管分叉处黏膜受损。

9. 吸痰:

（1）用非惯用手拇指按住控制口,惯用手拇指和食指左右旋转吸痰管,边吸边提。**依据**:吸引时间为 8～10 秒(不超过 15 秒)以减少氧耗。

（2）Withdraw the catheter completely, and stop suctioning.

（3）Hyperoxygenate the patient for 1-2 minutes between suctioning (or hyperventilate the patient 10-15 times using the Ambu bag). **Rationale**：*This provides an opportunity for reoxygenation of the lungs.*

10. Reassess the patient's oxygen saturation and repeat suctioning：

（1）Observe the patient's respiration and skin color.

（2）If necessary, take the patient's pulse.

（3）Encourage the patient to breathe deeply and cough between suctions.

（4）Flush the catheter and repeat suctioning until the airway is clear and the breathing is relatively effortless and quiet.

11. Dispose of the equipment：

（1）Flush the catheter and the tubing.

（2）Turn off the suction, disconnect the catheter, and insert the suction tubing adapter into an empty bottle (or wrap the adapter with a piece of sterile gauze). Wrap the catheter with the gloved hand and remove the glove so that it turns inside out over the catheter.

（3）Dispose of the used equipment appropriately.

（4）Use a new sterile catheter and a disposable sterile container for each suctioning. Empty and clean the suction collection container when it is 2/3 filled. Change other equipment daily.

12. Assess the effectiveness of suctioning: Auscultate the patient's breath sounds to ensure it is clear of secretions. Observe dyspnea, skin color and oxygen saturation level.

13. Assist the patient to take a position that helps breathing.

14. Perform hand hygiene.

15. Be sure that the oxygen flow is returned to the previous level after hyperoxygenating the patient for 1-2 minutes. **Rationale**：*It is very dangerous to keep the patient on 100% oxygen.*

（2）拔出吸痰管,停止吸引。

（3）吸痰间歇给予高流量吸氧1～2分钟(或用呼吸皮囊加压呼吸10～15次)。**依据**:可增加氧储备。

10. 再次评估病人的氧饱和度,重复吸痰：

（1）观察病人呼吸和皮肤颜色。

（2）必要时测脉搏。

（3）鼓励病人在吸痰间歇深呼吸及咳嗽。

（4）冲洗吸痰管,重复吸痰至气道通畅、呼吸较前改善、呼吸平稳。

11. 处理用物：

（1）吸痰完毕,冲洗吸痰管及橡胶导管。

（2）关闭吸引器开关,分离吸痰管。将橡胶导管末端插入空瓶中(或用无菌纱布包裹),手套内面向外翻转脱下,包裹吸痰管。

（3）合理处置用物。

（4）吸痰管、一次性无菌容器每次更换,痰液收集瓶至2/3满时应及时倾倒和清洗,其他用物每日更换。

12. 评估吸痰效果:听诊肺部,确定呼吸音已变清,观察呼吸困难情况、面色及氧饱和度。

13. 协助病人取利于呼吸的体位。

14. 洗手。

15. 高流量吸氧1～2分钟后将氧流量调至吸痰前水平。**依据**:吸入纯氧易致氧中毒。

16. Replenish the sterile supplies for the next use. **Rationale**：*Patients who require suctioning often require it quickly, so it is essential to leave the equipment at the bedside ready for use.*

17. Provide important instructions.

18. Document relevant data：the amount and character of sputum and any other relevant condition.

## EVALUATION

1. Evaluate the effectiveness of suctioning (e.g., respiratory rate, depth and rhythm, breath sounds, skin color, the character and amount of sputum, changes in the vital signs).

2. Report any abnormal findings to the doctor in charge.

16.补充下次吸痰所需用物。

**依据**:吸痰用物必须备齐放置床边,以便随时吸痰。

17.交代注意事项。

18.记录痰液量、性质及其他病情。

## 评价

1.评价吸痰效果(如呼吸频率、深度、节律、呼吸音、皮肤颜色、痰液性状和量、生命体征改变情况)。

2.如有异常情况,报告主管医生。

# Words and Expressions

accumulate *vt.* 积累,积聚

adapter *n.* 转接器,适配器

airway *n.* 气道

Ambu bag/resuscitator/resuscitation bag 加压给氧皮囊,呼吸皮囊

auscultate *v.* 听诊

bifurcation *n.* 分支,分叉

bubbling *adj.* 冒泡的,水泡的

copious *adj.* 很多的,大量的

expansion *n.* 扩张,膨胀

fraction of inspired oxygen（$FiO_2$）吸入氧浓度

gauge *n.* 测量仪表,计量器

goggles *n.* 护目镜,风镜,游泳镜

hyperoxygenate *vt.* 过度氧合

hyperventilate *vt.* 通气过度

hypoxemia *n.* 低氧血症

（后缀-emia 表示"血液"）

intermittent *adj.* 间歇的,断断续续的

occlude *vt.* 使闭塞,堵塞

pneumonia *n.* 肺炎

（前缀 pneum-/pneumo-,pneumon-/pneumono- 表示"空气,肺泡"）

portable *adj.* 便携式的,轻便的

replenish *vt.* 补充,重新装满

restrict *vt.* 限制,限定（数量、范围等）

resuscitation *n.* 复苏,复活

resuscitator *n.* 人工呼吸器

saturation *n.* 饱和,饱和度

semi-Fowler's position 半坐卧位（30°～45°角）

（前缀 semi- 表示"半,部分"）

shield *n.* 防护屏,保护物,屏障

sputum *n.* 痰

sputum trap 集痰器

tachypnea *n.* 呼吸急促,呼吸过速

tidal *adj.* 潮汐的,有潮的

trachea *n.* 气管

tracheal *adj.* 气管的

tracheostomy *n.* 气管造口术

（前缀 trache-/tracheo- 表示"气管";后缀-ostomy 表示"开口,造口"）

trap *n.* 容器

trauma *n.* 精神创伤,挫折

unobstructed *adj.* 畅通无阻的,没有阻碍的

withdraw *vt.* 抽吸,退出,提现

# SKILL 12　Administering Oxygen by Cannula or Face Mask

# 技能操作 12　鼻导管、面罩吸氧法

Administering oxygen is a common therapy for patients. It is prescribed by the doctor who specifies the concentration and method of delivery. The nurse needs to adjust the oxygen flow rate according to the patient's condition. Oxygen is not completely harmless to the patient. Excessive amount of oxygen may lead to oxygen toxicity. It is crucial for nurses to inform patients about safety precautions of oxygen therapy.

氧疗是一种常用的治疗方法，由医生开出医嘱，确定吸氧浓度和方法。护士需要根据病情调节氧流量。氧气对病人并非完全无害，过高的氧浓度可导致氧中毒。护士应指导病人安全用氧。

二维码 12-1

二维码 12-2

## PURPOSES

### Cannula

1. To deliver a relatively low flow rate of oxygen when minimal $O_2$ is required.

2. To allow continuous oxygen supply while the patient is ingesting food or fluids.

### Face Mask

● To provide moderate $O_2$ support and a higher concentration and/or humidity of oxygen than by the cannula.

## ASSESSMENT

1. Assess skin and mucous membrane color.

2. Assess the patient's consciousness and breathing pattern.

3. Assess the ability of cooperation.

4. Check nostrils for patency and intactness of the nasal tissues.

## 目的

### 鼻导管法

1. 为低流量氧气吸入者供氧。

2. 使病人摄入食物或液体时不中断吸氧。

### 面罩法

● 提供中等浓度氧疗，较鼻导管法提供更高浓度或湿度的氧气。

## 评估

1. 皮肤及黏膜颜色。

2. 意识、呼吸形态。

3. 合作程度。

4. 鼻腔是否通畅，鼻黏膜是否完整。

5. Assess history of nasal surgery and deviated septum.

6. Assess presence of clinical signs of hypoxemia: tachycardia, tachypnea, restlessness, dyspnea, cyanosis and confusion (tachycardia and tachypnea are often early signs while confusion is a later sign).

7. Check the results of arterial blood gases (ABG) analysis.

8. Identify whether the patient has COPD (chronic obstructive pulmonary disease). A high carbon dioxide level normally stimulates respiration. However, a patient with COPD have a chronically elevated carbon dioxide level which desensitizes the respiration center. Low oxygen concentration is the main stimulus for respiration for such patients. Thus, oxygen must be given at a low flow rate. During continuous oxygen therapy, testing arterial blood gas level of oxygen ($PaO_2$) and that of carbon dioxide ($PaCO_2$) periodically is necessary.

## PLANNING

### Equipment

**Single-prong nasal cannula**

1. Oxygen tank (see Figure 12-1) or wall oxygen supply (see Figure 12-1), with a flow meter (see Figure 12-1)
2. Oxygen in-pipe
3. Humidifier with distilled water or as prescribed
4. Single-prong nasal cannula
5. Cannula tubing and adapter
6. Wrench (if oxygen tank is used)
7. Kidney dish
8. Clean gauze
9. Safety pin and elastic band
10. Adhesive tape
11. Swabs
12. Clean water
13. Oxygen flow chart

5. 鼻部手术史、鼻中隔是否偏曲。

6. 缺氧的临床体征:心动过速、呼吸急促、不安、呼吸困难、发绀、意识模糊等(心动过速和呼吸急促通常为早期缺氧体征,而意识模糊为晚期缺氧体征)。

7. 动脉血气(ABG)分析结果。

8. 病人是否有 COPD(慢性阻塞性肺病)。血中高浓度的 $CO_2$ 能刺激呼吸中枢,但 COPD 病人动脉血二氧化碳分压($PaCO_2$)长期处于高水平,呼吸中枢已失去对 $CO_2$ 的敏感性。此时主要依赖缺氧刺激呼吸,故应给予病人低流量吸氧。在连续吸氧过程中,应定期检测动脉血氧分压($PaO_2$)及二氧化碳分压($PaCO_2$)。

## 计划

### 用物准备

**单侧鼻导管法**

1. 氧气筒(见图 12-1)或中心供氧源(见图 12-1),氧气表(见图 12-1)
2. 湿化管芯
3. 湿化瓶(内盛蒸馏水或遵医嘱)
4. 单侧鼻导管
5. 出气橡胶管,接管
6. 扳手(使用氧气筒时)
7. 弯盘
8. 清洁纱布
9. 别针,橡皮筋
10. 胶布
11. 棉签
12. 一杯清水
13. 流量观察卡

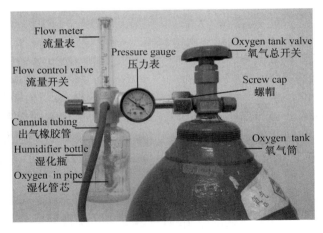

Figure 12-1    An oxygen tank with a flow meter

图 12-1    氧气筒及氧气表

### Nasal cannula

1. Oxygen supply with a flow meter

2. Humidifier with distilled water or as prescribed

3. Nasal cannula

4. Oxygen flow chart

### Face Mask

1. Oxygen supply with a flow meter

2. Humidifier with distilled water or as prescribed

3. Face mask of the proper size

4. Oxygen flow chart

## IMPLEMENTATION

### Preparation

• Fill 1/3-1/2 of the humidifier bottle with distilled water or as prescribed.

### Procedure

1. Perform hand hygiene, and put on a mask.

2. Before the procedure, introduce yourself and verify the patient's identity.

3. Explain to the patient the purpose of administering oxygen.

4. Protect the patient's privacy.

5. If possible, assist the patient to take a semi-

### 双侧鼻导管法

1.供氧装置,氧气表

2.湿化瓶(内盛蒸馏水或遵医嘱)

3.双侧鼻导管

4.流量观察卡

### 面罩法

1.供氧装置,氧气表

2.湿化瓶(内盛蒸馏水或遵医嘱)

3.型号合适的面罩

4.流量观察卡

## 实施

### 准备

• 湿化瓶中盛 1/3～1/2 蒸馏水或遵医嘱。

### 操作步骤

1.洗手,戴口罩。

2.操作前自我介绍并确认病人。

3.解释用氧目的。

4.保护病人隐私。

5.如病情允许,协助病人取

Fowler's position. **Rationale**：*This position permits easier chest expansion and hence easier breathing.*

6. Prepare adhesive tape. Clean the naris (nares) with wet swabs.

7. Set up the oxygen equipment and the humidifier：

(1) If an oxygen tank is to be used, clean the outlet of the tank (this can be done before approaching the bedside).

(2) Attach the flow meter to the tank (using a wrench to tighten the connection) or the wall outlet. The flow meter should be turned off.

(3) Turn on the oxygen, and the connections should be airtight.

(4) Attach the oxygen in-pipe and the humidifier to the base of the flow meter.

(5) Attach the cannula tubing to the flow meter, and connect the adapter to the cannula tubing.

8. Apply the appropriate oxygen device.

**Single-prong nasal cannula**

(1) Attach the single-prong nasal cannula to the tubing. There should be no kinks in the tubing, and the connections are airtight.

(2) Turn on the flow control valve, set the oxygen at the prescribed rate (see Figure 12-4), and ensure proper functioning.

(3) Place the tip of the cannula in water to check the oxygen flow and at the same time moisten the cannula tip.

(4) Measure the length which is 2/3 of the distance from the nostril to the earlobe (see Figure 12-5). Carefully insert the cannula into the selected nostril. Secure the tube by taping it to the nose and cheek with adhesive tape.

(5) Pin the cannula tubing to the shoulder of the patient's gown.

**Nasal cannula**

(1) Clean the nares with wet swabs.

(2) Connect the nasal cannula to oxygen flow meter directly.

半坐卧位。**依据**：半坐卧位使胸腔易于扩张,有利于呼吸。

6.准备胶布,用湿棉签清洁鼻腔。

7.装氧气表及湿化瓶：

(1)如使用氧气筒,先清洁气门(此步骤可于氧气筒推至病房前完成)。

(2)将氧气表连接至氧气筒(用扳手将螺旋拧紧)或中心供氧源。检查流量开关(应关闭)。

(3)打开氧气总开关,无漏气。

(4)连接氧气湿化管芯及湿化瓶。

(5)连接出气橡胶管及接管。

8.选择合适的吸氧用具。

**单侧鼻导管法**

(1)将单侧鼻导管与橡胶管相连,橡胶管无扭曲,各部分连接紧密。

(2)打开流量开关,调节氧流量(见图 12-4),确认氧气流出平稳。

(3)将鼻导管前端放入水杯中试气,同时润滑鼻导管。

(4)用鼻导管测量插入长度,为鼻尖到耳垂的 2/3 (见图 12-5)。动作轻柔地插入鼻导管,用胶布将鼻导管固定于鼻翼及面颊部。

(5)用别针将橡胶管固定于病人肩部衣服上。

**双侧鼻导管法**

(1)用湿棉签清洁两侧鼻腔。

(2)将双侧鼻导管直接连至氧气表。

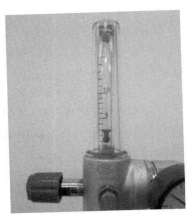

Figure 12-4    This flow rate is set to deliver 3L/min

图 12-4    流量调节至 3 L/min

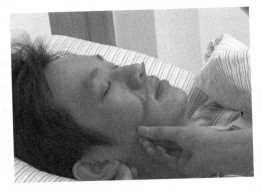

Figure 12-5    Measuring the length of the cannula inserted

图 12-5    测量鼻导管插入长度

（3）Place the outlets of the cannula in water to check the airflow.

（4）Fit the outlet prongs into the patient's nares, and both sides of the tubing hooked around the ears. Adjust the strap under the chin (see Figure 12-6).

（3）双侧鼻导管出气口放入水杯中试气。

（4）将出气口插入病人鼻孔，两侧导管沿双耳向下环绕，调节颏下导管松紧度（见图 12-6）。

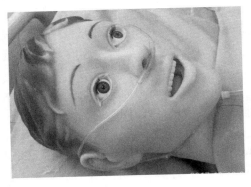

Figure 12-6    A nasal cannula

图 12-6    双侧鼻导管

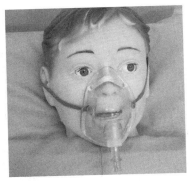

Figure 12-7    A simple face mask

图 12-7    简易面罩

**Face mask**

（1）Place the mask over the patient's face from the root of the nose downwards (see Figure 12-7). **Rationale**: *The mask should be nicely worn so that very little oxygen escapes.*

（2）Secure the elastic band around the patient's

**面罩法**

（1）将面罩从鼻根部向下罩于病人面部（见图 12-7）。**依据**：面罩须紧贴面部，减少氧气泄漏。

（2）松紧带环绕枕部使面罩

head so that the mask is snug and comfortable.

9. Inform the patient about the safety precautions of oxygen use.

10. Perform hand hygiene.

11. Document the relevant information.

12. Regularly assess the patient：

（1）Assess the patient in 15-30 minutes，then regularly thereafter，depending on the patient's condition.

（2）Assess the patient's vital signs，level of anxiety，skin color and breathing.

（3）Check if there are clinical signs of hypoxia，confusion，dyspnea，restlessness and cyanosis. Check ABG analysis results when available.

13. Inspect the equipment on a regular basis：

（1）Check the oxygen flow rate and the water volume in the humidifier every 30 minutes （and whenever providing care to the patient）.

（2）Make sure that safety precautions are being followed（keep away from fire，oil，heat sources and prevent shaking if an oxygen tank is used）.

**Stopping oxygen therapy**

1. Carry the equipment to the bedside.

2. Perform hand hygiene，and put on a mask.

3. Before performing the procedure，introduce yourself and verify the patient's identity. Explain to the patient the reason for stopping oxygen therapy.

4. Protect the patient's privacy.

5. Unpin the cannula tubing from the patient's gown，gently remove the adhesive tape，remove the cannula and wipe the nose with a piece of gauze.

6. Dispose of the cannula in the trash bag.

7. Turn off the oxygen tank valve，release the remaining oxygen in the flow meter，then turn off the flow control valve.

8. Disconnect the cannula tubing，humidifier and oxygen in-pine from the oxygen flow meter.

9. Dispose of the used equipment appropriately.

服帖舒适。

9. 指导病人安全用氧。

10. 洗手。

11. 记录。

12. 定期评估病人：

（1）吸氧15～30分钟后评估病人，之后根据病情定期评估。

（2）评估病人生命体征、情绪、皮肤颜色及呼吸状况。

（3）观察病人有无缺氧体征、意识模糊、呼吸困难、不安和发绀的临床表现，查看 ABG 分析结果。

13. 定期检查吸氧装置：

（1）每30分钟（以及每次护理病人时）检查氧流量及湿化瓶中的水量。

（2）确保用氧安全（"防火、防油、防热，用氧气瓶还应防震"）。

**停氧**

1. 携用物至床旁。

2. 洗手，戴口罩。

3. 操作前自我介绍并确认病人。向病人解释停氧原因。

4. 保护病人隐私。

5. 取下别针，轻轻揭去胶布，拔出鼻导管，用纱布擦净鼻部。

6. 将鼻导管置入垃圾袋。

7. 关氧气总开关，放出余氧，关上流量开关。

8. 取下橡胶管、湿化瓶和湿化管芯。

9. 合理弃置用物。

10. Using a wrench, loosen the screw connecting the flow meter and oxygen tank. Disconnect the flow meter.

11. Assist the patient to take a comfortable position, and provide relevant instructions.

12. Perform hand hygiene.

13. Record the time of stopping oxygen therapy and the patient's reaction.

## EVALUATION

1. Evaluate the effectiveness of oxygen therapy.

2. Report any abnormal findings to the doctor in charge after removing the oxygen.

10. 用扳手松开连接氧气表和氧气筒的螺旋，取下氧气表。

11. 协助病人躺卧舒适，交代注意事项。

12. 洗手。

13. 记录停氧时间及病人反应。

## 评价

1. 评价吸氧效果。

2. 停氧后如病情出现较大变化，报告主管医生。

# Words and Expressions

arterial blood gases（ABG）analysis 动脉血气分析

adhesive *adj.* 黏的，黏附的

airtight *adj.* 不透气的，密封的

cannula *n.*（输液等的）套管，插管

carbon *n.* 碳

carbon dioxide（$CO_2$）二氧化碳

chronic *adj.*（尤指疾病）慢性的，长期的

chronic obstructive pulmonary disease（COPD）慢性阻塞性肺疾病

chronically *adv.* 长期地，慢性地

confusion *n.* 混淆，困惑

deviate *vt.* 偏离

dioxide *n.* 二氧化物

（前缀 di- 表示"两次，两倍"）

earlobe *n.* 耳垂

humidifier *n.* 加湿器，增湿器

humidity *n.* 湿度

hypoxia *n.* 低氧，缺氧

kink *n.* 结；*vi.* 使扭结

nares *n.* 鼻孔（naris 的复数）

nasal *adj.* 鼻的

（前缀 nas-/naso- 表示"鼻"）

arterial partial carbon dioxide pressure（$PaCO_2$）动脉血二氧化碳分压

arterial partial oxygen pressure（$PaO_2$）动脉血氧分压

prescribe *vt.* 给……开（药），开（处方）

prescription *n.* 药方，处方

prong *n.* 叉子齿，叉齿

pulmonary *adj.* 肺的，肺部的

septum *n.* 隔膜

snug *adj.* 贴身的，严实的

strap *n.* 带子；*vt.* 用带子系好

toxicity *n.* 毒性，毒力

tachycardia *n.* 心动过速，心跳过速

（前缀 tachy- 表示"快速，加速"；后缀 -cardia 表示"心脏跳动"）

wrench *n.* 扳手，扳钳

# SKILL 13    Inserting a Nasogastric Tube and Administering Tube Feeding

# 技能操作 13
# 插鼻胃管及
# 鼻饲法

A nasogastric (NG) tube is used to ensure adequate nutrition intake in patients who can not swallow food, or suction gastric contents or provide treatment for patients whose upper gastrointestinal (GI) tract is impaired and in whom the transport of food to the small intestine is interrupted. Inserting an NG tube is an invasive procedure. Nurses need to apply knowledge (e. g., anatomy, physiology, risk prevention and communication skills) so as to avoid unnecessary damage to the digestive tract and to solve any problem that might occur during insertion.

胃管插入可供给不能经口进食的病人足够的营养,对胃肠梗阻病人进行胃肠减压或进行治疗。插胃管是一项侵入性操作,护士需运用所学知识(如解剖学、生理学、风险防范知识和沟通技巧)进行插管,防止不必要的消化道黏膜损伤,并能妥善处理插管过程中可能出现的问题。

二维码 13-1

二维码 13-2

## PURPOSES

1. To maintain the nutritional status for patients who are unable to eat for some reasons (e. g., unconsciousness, oral diseases or after oral surgery, dysphagia, being unable to open mouth).

2. To administer medications.

## ASSESSMENT

1. Assess the patient's mental status and ability to cooperate.

2. Ask the patient about his/her experiences of NG tube insertion.

3. Using a flashlight, observe the intactness of the nasal tissues.

4. Examine the nares for any obstruction or deformity by asking the patient to breathe through one nostril while occluding the other.

## 目的

1. 维持因某些原因不能经口进食病人的营养(如昏迷、口腔疾患或口腔手术后、吞咽困难、不能张口者)。

2. 提供药物。

## 评估

1. 评估病人的精神状态及合作能力。

2. 询问病人有无插胃管史。

3. 用手电筒观察鼻腔黏膜是否完好。

4. 嘱病人按压一侧鼻腔,用另一侧鼻腔呼吸以检查有无鼻腔阻塞或畸形。

5. Select the nostril which has the greater airflow.

5．选择较通畅侧鼻腔插管。

## PLANNING

### Equipment

1. Nasogastric tube of the proper size
2. Adhesive tape
3. Liquid paraffin
4. Kidney dish
5. Disposable pad/towel
6. Stethoscope
7. 50-mL syringe
8. Swabs
9. Safety pin and elastic band
10. Flashlight
11. Liquid formula
12. Warm water
13. Plain tissue forceps
14. Feeding set and IV pole if the feeding bag (bottle) is used
15. Sticky label for NG tube
16. Clean bowl
17. Clean gloves
18. Facial tissues

## IMPLEMENTATION

### Preparation

1. Check the expiration date of the feeding formula.
2. Organize the equipment.

### Procedure

**Inserting an NG Tube**

1. Carry the equipment to the bedside. Before performing the procedure, introduce yourself and verify the patient's identity. Explain to the patient or the family what you are going to do, why it is necessary and how he/she can cooperate. Insertion of the tube is uncomfortable. Make an agreement for the patient to indicate sick and a desire for stopping the insertion. Raising a hand is

## 计划

### 用物准备

1．型号适合的胃管
2．胶布
3．液体石蜡
4．弯盘
5．一次性护理垫/毛巾
6．听诊器
7．50 mL 注射器
8．棉签
9．别针、橡皮筋
10．手电筒
11．鼻饲液
12．温开水
13．无齿镊
14．如用营养袋(瓶),准备鼻饲输注器及输液架
15．胃管标签贴
16．清洁碗
17．清洁手套
18．面巾纸

## 实施

### 准备

1．检查鼻饲液的有效期。
2．备齐用物。

### 操作步骤

**插鼻胃管法**

1．携用物至床旁,操作前自我介绍,确认病人。向病人或家属解释操作内容、目的和配合方法。插胃管通常引起不适,当病人感觉难受需要暂停时,可让病人举手示意。

often used for this purpose.

2. Protect privacy by drawing the curtains around the bed or closing the door of the room.

3. Remove dentures, if present.

4. Prepare the patient's position：

(1) If the patient's condition permits, assist him/her to take a sitting or high-Fowler's position. **Rationale**：*It is easier for patients to swallow in these two positions and gravity helps the insertion of the tube.*

(2) If the patient is unable to sit, position the patient on his/her right lateral position.

(3) For unconscious patients, remove the pillow and hyperextend the patient's neck backwards.

5. Perform hand hygiene, and put on a mask.

6. Place a disposable pad across the chest, under the chin. Place a kidney dish near the mouth.

7. Clean the selected nostril with a wet swab.

8. Prepare adhesive tape, open the syringe, and pour a small amount of liquid paraffin into the clean bowl to soak the gauze.

9. Wear clean gloves.

10. Measure the length of the tube to be inserted：

(1) Use the tube to measure the distance from the nasal tip to the earlobe and then from the earlobe to the xiphoid process (see Figure 13-1), or from the hairline to the xiphoid process (see Figure 13-2). **Rationale**：*This length approximates the distance from the nares to the stomach. This distance varies among individuals.* Generally, 45-55 cm is appropriate for adults.

(2) Note the length of the tube to be inserted (or mark this length with a piece of adhesive tape if the tube does not have scale).

11. Insert the tube：

(1) Lubricate the tip of the tube with liquid paraffin.

2.拉上床边围帘或关门以保护病人隐私。

3.有义齿者取下义齿。

4.病人体位准备：

(1)如病情允许,协助病人取坐位或高半坐卧位。**依据**：此两种体位利于病人吞咽及借重力作用使胃管易于插入。

(2)无法坐起者取右侧卧位。

(3)协助昏迷病人取去枕仰卧位,头后仰。

5.洗手,戴口罩。

6.铺一次性护理垫于胸前颏下,置弯盘于口角旁。

7.用湿棉签清洁鼻腔。

8.准备胶布及注射器,倒少许液体石蜡于清洁碗中浸湿纱布。

9.戴清洁手套。

10.测量胃管插入长度：

(1)插入长度为由鼻尖经耳垂至胸骨剑突(见图13-1)或从前额发际至胸骨剑突的距离(见图13-2)。**依据**：此长度相当于从鼻孔到胃的距离,有个体差异。一般成人插入长度为45～55 cm。

(2)标记插入长度(如胃管无刻度,用一小条胶布做标识)。

11.插管：

(1)用液体石蜡纱布润滑胃管前端。

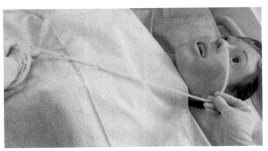

Figure 13-1　Measuring the length of the NG tube to be inserted（nasal tip—earlobe—xiphoid process）

图 13-1　测量鼻胃管插入长度（鼻尖—耳垂—剑突）

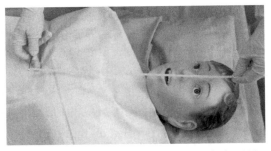

Figure 13-2　Measuring the length of the NG tube to be inserted（from hairline to the xiphoid process）

图 13-2　测量鼻胃管插入长度（前额发际线至剑突）

（2）Ask her/her to extend his/her head back and gently insert the tube from the selected nostril towards the nasopharynx. **Rationale**：*Hyperextension of the neck reduces the curvature of the nasopharyngeal junction.*

（3）Once the tube reaches the oropharynx（throat）, it may cause nausea. Some patients' eyes may water at this point. **Rationale**：*Tears are a natural body response. Wipe away tears with tissues for the patient.* Ask the patient to swallow.

（4）If resistance is felt, withdraw the tube a little, then advance it again. **Rationale**：*The tube should never be forced against resistance because of the danger of injury.*

（5）If the patient vomits, stop inserting the tube temporarily, and allow the patient to rest for a while and to take a few deep breaths or sips of warm water. **Rationale**：*Swallowing moves the epiglottis over the opening to the larynx.*

（6）If the patient continues to gag and the tube can not advance with each swallow, inspect the mouth. **Rationale**：*The tube may be coiled in the mouth. If so, withdraw it until it is straight, and try again to carefully insert it.*

（7）If the tube mistakenly goes into the airway, immediately withdraw it and allow the patient to rest for a while, then insert it again.

（2）嘱病人头尽量向后仰，动作轻柔地将胃管从鼻腔插向鼻咽部。**依据**：头后仰可使鼻咽部通道变直。

（3）当胃管插到咽喉部时，可引起恶心，甚至眼泪流出。**依据**：插管引起流泪为机体自然反应，协助病人用纸巾擦干。嘱病人做吞咽动作。

（4）如插管时遇到阻力，可将胃管抽出少许再插。**依据**：不可强行插管以免损伤食管黏膜。

（5）如出现呕吐，应暂停插管，让病人休息片刻，嘱病人深呼吸或喝少量温开水。**依据**：吞咽时会厌软骨盖住喉入口。

（6）如病人持续恶心，胃管不能随吞咽动作插入时，应检查口腔。**依据**：胃管可能盘曲在口腔中；如是，将其拔出捋直。

（7）如胃管不慎误入气管，应立即拔出，让病人休息片刻后重新插入。

(8) With the patient's cooperation，continue inserting for 5-10 cm with each swallow until the indicated length is achieved.

(9) For an unconscious patient，when the tube is inserted for about 15 cm，elevate his/her head，bring the lower jaw close to the manubrium of sternum with your non-dominant hand and continue inserting the tube slowly with your dominant hand.

12. Secure the tube by taping it to the nose.

13. Make sure the gastric tube is in the stomach：

(1) Gastric contents can be aspirated with a syringe.

(2) Gurgling sounds can be heard with a stethoscope placed over the patient's epigastrium while injecting 10mL of air quickly into the stomach through the tube.

(3) There is no air bubble coming out when the end of the tube is put in water.

14. Administer the liquid formula：

Ensure the appropriate temperature（38-40 ℃）of the liquid before administration. It is advisable to test the temperature of the liquid on the inner part of the wrist without feeling hot.

▶Syringe（closed system）

(1) Withdraw 20～30 mL of warm water into a syringe，connect the syringe to the NG tube and inject warm water slowly through the tube.

(2) Pinch the tube before disconnecting the syringe each time，withdraw 50 mL of the liquid formula and inject it through the NG tube slowly（see Figure 13-3）. After finishing feeding（≤200 mL），flush the tube by injecting 20～30 mL of warm water in a pulsed manner. **Rationale**：*Water flushing prevents the tube from being blocked with sticky liquid*.

(3) Disconnect the syringe and raise the tube to allow the water to flow down through the tube. Plug the tube before the water is drained out in the tube.

▶Syringe（open system）

(1) Remove the plunger from the syringe and connect the syringe to a pinched or clamped tube（see Figure 13-4）.

（8）在病人的配合下，每吞咽一次插入 5～10 cm，直至预定长度。

（9）为昏迷病人插管至10～15 cm 时，用非惯用手将其头部托起，使下颏靠近胸骨柄，同时另一手持镊子将胃管慢慢插入。

12. 用胶布将胃管固定在鼻翼。

13. 确认胃管在胃内的方法：

（1）胃管末端连接注射器，能抽到胃液。

（2）置听诊器于病人上腹部，快速经胃管向胃内注入 10 mL 空气，听到气过水声。

（3）将胃管末端放入水杯中，无气泡逸出。

14. 灌注鼻饲液：

鼻饲液温度适宜（38～40 ℃），可用手腕掌侧测试鼻饲液温度，以感觉不烫为宜。

▶注射器法（密闭式）

（1）注射器内抽取 20～30 mL 温开水，接至胃管末端，缓慢注入温开水。

（2）每次取下注射器前捏住胃管。抽取 50 mL 鼻饲液，从胃管缓慢注入（见图 13-3）。鼻饲完毕（≤200 mL），脉冲式注入 20～30 mL 温开水冲洗胃管。**依据**：温开水冲洗防止胃管被黏稠食物堵塞。

（3）取下注射器，抬高胃管使温开水流入胃内，温开水流尽前塞住胃管末端。

▶注射器法（开放式）

（1）拔出注射器活塞，胃管末端连接注射器空筒（见图 13-4）。

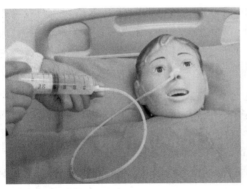

Figure 13-3　Using a syringe to administer tube feeding

图 13-3　注射器空筒法(开放式)鼻饲

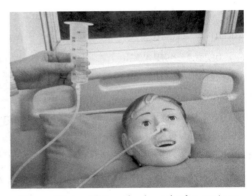

Figure 13-4　Using the barrel of a syringe to administer tube feeding

图 13-4　注射器注射法(密闭式)鼻饲

（2）Slowly pour the liquid formula into the syringe barrel，and allow it to flow down by gravity. Raise or lower the barrel to adjust the flow rate as needed. Pinch or clamp the tubing for a minute if the patient feels uncomfortable.

（3）When finishing feeding，pour 20～30 mL of warm water into the syringe barrel before the syringe is empty.

（4）Disconnect the syringe before warm water is drained out in the NG tube and plug the tube.

▶Feeding bag

（1）Check the label of the feeding bag for the expiration date of the liquid formula.

（2）Expose the insertion site of the bag by removing the protective cover.

（3）Ensure the sterility of the feeding infusion set before opening the package, close the clamp of the tubing, remove the cap from the spike and insert the spike into the insertion site of the feeding bag (bottle).

（4）Hang the feeding bag (bottle) on the IV pole, squeeze the drip chamber until it is one third to one half filled with the liquid formula.

（5）Turn on the clamp, and have the liquid run through the tubing to remove the air in the tubing. Reclamp the tubing, attach the feeding tubing to the NG tube, and turn on the clamp to start feeding (a

（2）缓慢将鼻饲液倒入注射器空筒，借重力作用使其流入胃内，通过抬高或降低注射器空筒调节流速。如病人感觉不适，可捏住或夹住管子，暂停片刻。

（3）鼻饲完毕，注射器空筒内鼻饲液流尽前倒入 20～30 mL 温开水。

（4）胃管内温开水流尽前取下注射器空筒，塞住胃管。

▶营养袋鼻饲法

（1）查看营养袋标签，确定鼻饲液在有效期内。

（2）除去营养袋插口的保护套。

（3）确定输注器有效后打开包装，夹闭调节器，去掉输注器插头保护套后插入营养袋（瓶）插口。

（4）挂营养袋（瓶）于输液架上，挤压茂菲氏滴管使液面达滴管的 1/3～1/2 满。

（5）打开调节器，排尽管内空气后与胃管相连，打开调节器开始鼻饲（在重症病房，通常使用营养泵以准确控制滴速）。

flow-control device or feeding pump is generally used to provide an accurate flow rate in the acute health care settings).

（6）Apply a label on the set just below the chamber to differentiate with other tubes.

（7）When finishing feeding，disconnect the feeding tubing from the NG tube.

（8）Flush the NG tube in a pulsed manner with 20～30 mL of warm water using a syringe every 4 hours and when finishing feeding.

15. Remove and discard the gloves.

16. Remove the pad and kidney dish.

17. Secure the tube to the patient's cheek with adhesive tape.

18. Wrap the end of the NG tube with a piece of gauze and fold it with an elastic band around it. Pin the end of the tube to the gown （shoulder part）.
**Rationale**：*This prevents the tube from dangling and pulling.*

19. Perform hand hygiene.

20. Apply a label on the NG tube，indicating the name of the tube，the date and length of the tube inserted.

21. Ensure the patient's comfort and safety：ask the patient to remain this position for at least 30 minutes.

22. Dispose of the equipment appropriately：

（1）If the equipment is to be reused，wash it thoroughly with clean water so that it is ready to reuse.

（2）Change the equipment every 24 hours.

23. Perform hand hygiene.

24. Document relevant information：

（1）Record the amount and kind of the fluid administered （including the liquid formula and warm water used to flush the tubing），duration of the feeding，and the patient's assessment results.

（2）Document the volume of liquid formula and warm water in the patient's intake and output chart.

25. Monitor the patient for possible adverse reactions.

（6）在输注器滴管下方贴非静脉标签以区别于其他管道。

（7）鼻饲完毕,分离输注器和胃管。

（8）每 4 小时及鼻饲完毕时,用注射器抽取 20～30 mL 温开水以脉冲式冲洗胃管。

15. 脱下手套、弃置。

16. 撤去一次性护理垫和弯盘。

17. 用胶布将胃管固定于面颊部。

18. 用纱布包裹胃管末端并反折,用橡皮筋扎紧,用别针将胃管固定于病人肩部衣服上。**依据:**防止胃管摆晃及拔出。

19. 洗手。

20. 在胃管上贴标签,注明管道名称、插管日期和插入长度。

21. 确保病人舒适安全:嘱病人保持半卧位至少 30 分钟。

22. 合理处置用物:

（1）用清水洗净可重复使用的物品,备用。

（2）用物每 24 小时更换一次。

23. 洗手。

24. 记录:

（1）记录鼻饲液量和种类(鼻饲液和温开水的总量)、鼻饲时间、病人反应。

（2）将鼻饲液和温开水剂量记录在病人出入液量记录单上。

25. 观察可能出现的不良反应。

**Removing an NG tube**

1. Before the procedure, introduce yourself and verify the patient's identity. Explain to the patient the reason for removing the tube.

2. Perform hand hygiene, and put on a mask.

3. Protect the patient's privacy.

4. Unpin the tube from the patient's gown.

5. Place a disposable pad across the chest, under the chin. Place a kidney dish near the mouth.

6. Wear gloves.

7. Administer the last feeding before removing the tube:

(1) Attach the syringe to the end of the NG tube and aspirate gastric contents (this must be done before each feeding).

(2) If the tube is placed in the stomach, aspirate all contents and measure the amount of the residual every 4-6 hours.

(3) If >150 mL of the gastric contents is withdrawn, refer to the doctor in charge before proceeding.

**Or:**

1. Inject the gastric contents back into the stomach and flush 20~30 mL of warm water through the tubing, then administer feeding (the patient's position and feeding procedure are the same as previously described).

2. Clamp or pinch the end of the NG tube after feeding.

3. Gently remove the adhesive tape.

4. Ask the patient to take a deep breath, and remove the tube smoothly while the patient exhales. Wipe the nose with a piece of gauze.

5. Place the tube in the trash bag.

6. Ensure the patient's comfort:

(1) Assist the patient to rinse the mouth, then wipe the mouth with tissues.

(2) Assist the patient to blow the nose if needed. Wipe the face, especially where the adhesive tape was attached.

**拔胃管法**

1.操作前自我介绍,确认病人。向病人解释拔管原因。

2.洗手,戴口罩。

3.保护病人隐私。

4.取下别针。

5.铺一次性护理垫于胸前颏下,置弯盘于口角旁。

6.戴清洁手套。

7.拔管前鼻饲:

(1)注射器接胃管末端,有胃容物抽出(每次鼻饲前必须证实胃管在胃内)。

(2)留置胃管者应每4~6小时抽吸胃内容物一次以检查胃内潴留量。

(3)如潴留量>150 mL,应暂停鼻饲,报告主管医生。

**否则:**

1.将抽出的胃内容物注回胃内,再注入20~30 mL温开水以润滑胃管。病人体位、鼻饲程序同前。

2.鼻饲后捏紧或塞住胃管末端。

3.轻轻揭去胶布。

4.嘱病人深呼吸,在病人呼气时轻稳地拔出胃管,用纱布擦净鼻部。

5.弃置胃管。

6.保证病人舒适:

(1)协助病人漱口,用纸巾擦干口周。

(2)必要时协助病人擤鼻,擦脸,尤其是胶布粘贴处。

（3）Ask the patient to keep this position for at least 30 minutes.

7. Remove the pad and kidney dish. Dispose of the equipment appropriately.

8. Remove and discard the gloves.

9. Perform hand hygiene.

10. Record the time of removing the tube and the patient's reaction.

## EVALUATION

1. Observe the patient's reaction after the tube was removed (e. g. , nausea, vomiting), and check intactness of the nostrils.

2. Report to the doctor in charge if significant deviations occur.

（3）嘱病人维持该体位至少 30 分钟。

7. 撤去护理垫和弯盘,清理用物。

8. 脱下手套、弃置。

9. 洗手。

10. 记录拔管时间及病人反应。

## 评价

1. 观察拔管后病人的反应（有无恶心、呕吐）,检查鼻黏膜是否完好。

2. 如有异常情况,报告主管医师。

## Words and Expressions

anatomy *n.* 解剖,解剖学

barrel *n.* 枪管,桶

bubble *n.* 气泡

chamber *n.* 室,腔

curvature *n.* 弯曲,曲度

digestive *adj.* 消化的

dysphagia *n.* 吞咽困难

epigastrium *n.* 上腹部

　（前缀 epi- 表示"在 …… 上面,在 ……
　外面"）

epiglottis *n.* 会厌

formula *n.* 配方,处方

gag *vi.* 作呕;*n.* 塞口物

gastric *adj.* 胃的,胃部的

gastrointestinal(GI) *adj.* 胃肠的

gastrointestinal tract 消化道

gurgling *n.* 汩汩声的

hairline *n.*（尤指前额的）发际线

high-Fowler's position 高半坐卧位（60°～
　90°角）

hyperextend *vt.* 使……过度伸展

hyperextension *n.* 过度伸展

interrupt *vt.* 打断,打扰,打岔

intestine *n.* 肠

invasive *adj.* 侵入的,侵袭的

jaw *n.* 颌,下巴

junction *n.* 交叉点,接合点

manubrium *n.* 柄状体

nasogastric(NG) *adj.* 鼻胃的

nasopharyngeal *adj.* 鼻咽的

nausea *n.* 恶心,反胃

oropharynx *n.* 口咽

plunger *n.* 活塞

physiology *n.* 生理学

pulsed *adj.* 脉冲的;*v.* 使跳动

residual *adj.* 剩余的,残留的

spike *n.* 尖状物,尖头

sternum *n.* 胸骨

sticky *adj.* 黏（性）的

stomach *n.* 胃,腹部

xiphoid *n.* 剑状突起,剑状软骨

xiphoid process 剑突

# SKILL 14　Indwelling Urinary Catheterization

Urinary catheterization is usually performed only when it is absolutely necessary. The incidence of urinary tract infection(UTI) caused by indwelling urethral catheters is 70%-80%. The risk of infection increases by about 5 percentage points for each day that a catheter remains in place. Another hazard is trauma caused by urethral catheterization, particularly in the male patients. It is important to strictly follow the principle of aseptic techniques, insert the catheter at the correct angle, and avoid forcing the catheter to get in.

二维码 14-1

## CLINICAL ALERTS

1. Use aseptic techniques and sterile equipment strictly.

2. Choose the catheter of the proper size, and insert the catheter gently to decrease urethral trauma.

3. Prevent the catheter and the tubing from kinking to keep urine flow smoothly.

4. Keep the urine bag below the bladder at all times, but avoid the urine bag touching the floor.

5. Empty the urine bag timely.

6. If the catheter is mistakenly inserted into the patient's vagina, use a new sterile catheter.

7. For a frail patient with a fully distended bladder, do not empty more than 1000 mL of urine for the first time to avoid collapse and hematuria.

# 技能操作 14 留置导尿术

导尿通常在病情必需时进行。留置导尿管引发尿路感染的发生率为 70%～80%，导尿管每留置一天，感染率增加约 5 个百分点。另外，插管还可引起尿道损伤，尤其是男性病人。因此，在操作时应严格遵守无菌操作原则，掌握正确的插管角度，避免强行插管。

二维码 14-2

## 注意事项

1. 严格执行无菌操作技术，使用无菌物品。

2. 选择型号合适的导尿管，插管动作轻柔以减少尿道黏膜损伤。

3. 防止导尿管和引流管扭曲，保持尿液引流通畅。

4. 始终保持集尿袋低于膀胱水平，避免集尿袋触及地面。

5. 及时排空集尿袋中尿液。

6. 若导尿管误入阴道，应更换导尿管。

7. 膀胱高度膨胀而极度虚弱的病人，第一次放尿不得超过1000mL，避免病人发生虚脱和血尿。

## PURPOSES

### Intermittent catheterization

1. To relieve discomfort due to bladder distention.

2. To assess the amount of residual urine if the bladder empties incompletely.

3. To collect a sterile urine specimen.

### Indwelling catheterization

1. To measure urine output for critically ill patients to monitor his/her condition.

2. To keep the bladder empty during a pelvic surgery to avoid accidental injury to the bladder.

3. To provide continuous bladder drainage or irrigation.

4. To avoid urine contaminating the incision after perineum surgery.

## ASSESSMENT

1. Based on the purpose，determine the most appropriate method of catheterization and the size of the catheter.

2. Assess the patient's condition. Determine the total amount of urine to be removed one time.

3. Assess the patient's consciousness and mental status and the ability of cooperation.

4. Assess the patient's perineum condition. Palpate the bladder to check for distension.

## PLANNING

### Equipment

1. Clean gloves
2. Supplies for catheterization：
（1）Bath towel
（2）A disposable catheterization set，containing：
1）Waterproof drape
2）Gloves
3）Kidney dishes

## 目的

### 一次性导尿术

1．为尿潴留病人引流出尿液，以减轻痛苦。

2．为排尿不尽病人测量残余尿量。

3．收集无菌尿标本。

### 留置导尿术

1．测量危重病人尿量以监测病情变化。

2．盆腔手术过程中使膀胱保持空虚状态，避免术中误伤。

3．便于持续膀胱引流或冲洗。

4．避免尿液污染会阴部手术切口。

## 评估

1．根据导尿目的确定适合的导尿方法及导尿管型号。

2．评估病情，确定一次可导出的尿量。

3．评估病人意识、心理状态及合作程度。

4．评估病人会阴部情况，检查膀胱充盈度。

## 计划

### 用物准备

1．清洁手套
2．导尿用物：
（1）浴巾
（2）一次性导尿包，内有：
1）一次性护理垫
2）手套
3）弯盘

4）Cotton balls soaked with antiseptic solution

5）Plain tissue forceps

6）Cotton balls soaked with liquid paraffin

7）Urine specimen container

8）10-mL syringe prefilled with sterile water

9）Foley catheter（see Figure 14-1）

10）Collection bag and the tubing

11）Gauze squares

12）Sticky label for the urinary catheter

（3）A sterile plastic straight catheter can be used for intermittent catherization（see Figure 14-2）

4）消毒液棉球

5）无齿镊（平镊）

6）液体石蜡棉球

7）尿标本容器

8）10 mL 载水注射器（已抽好灭菌用水）

9）气囊导尿管（见图 14-1）

10）集尿袋及导管

11）纱布块

12）导尿管标签贴

（3）一次性导尿可用无菌一次性导尿管（见图 14-2）

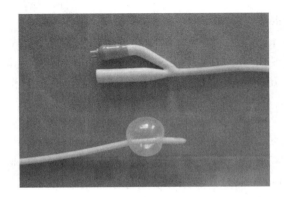

Figure 14-1　An indwelling（Foley）catheter
图 14-1　留置导尿管

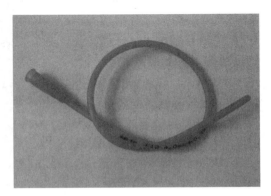

Figure 14-2　A straight urinary catheter
图 14-2　一次性使用导尿管

## IMPLEMENTATION

### Preparation

1. Ask the patient to clean his/her perineum. Perform routine perineal care for dependent patients with clean gloves.

2. Remove and discard the gloves.

3. Perform hand hygiene.

### Procedure

1. Before performing the procedure, introduce yourself and verify the patient's identity. Explain to the patient what you are going to do, why it is necessary, and how they can participate.

2. Perform hand hygiene and put on a mask.

## 实施

### 准备

1. 嘱病人清洗外阴。如病人不能自理，则护士戴清洁手套为其进行常规会阴护理。

2. 脱下手套，弃置。

3. 洗手。

### 操作步骤

1. 操作前自我介绍并确认病人，向病人解释操作内容、目的和配合方法。

2. 洗手，戴口罩。

3. Protect the patient's privacy.

4. Place the patient in an appropriate position. Take off the opposite trouser leg, cover it and a bath towel on the near leg. Drape the opposite leg with the quilt, and expose the perineum.

（1）Female：Take a supine position with knees flexed, feet apart for about 50-60 cm, thighs apart.

（2）Male：Take a supine position, thighs slightly apart.

5. Provide sufficient light. Stand on the patient's right side if you are right-handed, and stand on the patient's left side if you are left-handed.

6. Check the validity of the catheterization set.

7. Open the set and place it between the patient's thighs. Place a waterproof drape under the buttocks. Put the kidney dish near the perineum, and open the package of cutton balls. Wear a glove on your non-dominant hand.

8. Cleanse the perineum.

（1）Female：

Using tissue forceps, pick up a cutton ball with your dominant hand and wipe the perineal area orderly from top to bottom, from outside to inside. Wipe the mons pubis, opposite side of the labia majora and then the near side. Use the non-dominant hand to separate the labia majora and cleanse the labia minora in the same order. Finally, wipe carefully over the urethral meatus, then down to the anus (see Figure 14-3).

3. 保护病人隐私。

4. 协助病人取合适体位。脱去对侧裤腿，盖在近侧腿上，并盖上浴巾，对侧腿部用盖被遮盖。暴露外阴方法如下：

（1）女性病人：仰卧屈膝，两脚分开 50～60 cm，两腿外展。

（2）男性病人：仰卧，两腿稍外展。

5. 光线充足。操作者如是右撇子，则站在病人右侧，若是左撇子，则站病人左侧。

6. 检查导尿包有效期。

7. 打开导尿包放在病人两腿间，取出一次性护理垫，铺于臀下。将弯盘放在近会阴处，取出消毒液棉球。非惯用手戴清洁手套。

8. 初步消毒。

（1）女性病人：

操作者一手持镊子夹取消毒液棉球，自上而下、由外向内消毒外阴。先消毒阴阜、对侧大阴唇、近侧大阴唇，另一戴手套的手分开大阴唇，同法消毒小阴唇，最后消毒尿道口，擦至肛门口（见图14-3）。

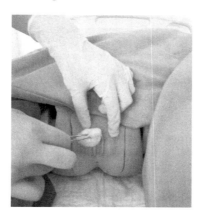

Figure 14-3　Cleansing the labia

图 14-3　消毒阴唇

(2) Male：

Using tissue forceps，pick up a cutton ball with your dominant hand. First wipe the mons pubis，then the penis and the scrotum. Use your non-dominant (gloved) hand to hold the penis with a piece of gauze just below the glans. If needed，push back the foreskin. Hold the penis firmly upright with slight tension and wipe the center of the meatus，the glans penis，then down to the coronal sulcus in a circular motion.

9. Always use a new cotton ball to clean one area. After cleansing，remove the glove，place it into the kidney dish and move the dish to the end of the bed.

10. Open the catheterization set completely using aseptic techniques. Wear sterile gloves.

11. Place the fenestrated drape over the perineum，and expose the urinary meatus.

12. Open all packages：

(1) Open the urine collection bag，straighten the tubing and ensure the bag is intact.

(2) Open the other packages and take out all supplies.

(3) Attach the prefilled syringe to the indwelling catheter，and check the balloon for air leak.

(4) Attach the catheter to the urine bag.

(5) Lubricate the catheter tip 2.5-5 cm for females，15-17.5 cm for males.

13. Cleanse the meatus again.

(1) Female：

Separate the labia minora with the non-dominant hand to fully expose the meatus. With the tissue forceps in your dominant hand，pick up a cleansing cotton ball. Wipe the meatus，then both sides of the labia minora. Lastly，wipe the urethral meatus again with a new cotton ball.

(2) Male：

Hold the penis with the non-dominant hand as mentioned before. With the forceps in your dominant hand，pick up a cleansing cotton ball. Wipe from the center of the

（2）男性病人：

操作者一手持镊子夹取消毒液棉球按阴阜、阴茎、阴囊的顺序进行消毒，另一戴手套的手取纱布裹住阴茎将包皮向后推，暴露尿道口，稍加用力，上提阴茎。自尿道口向外向后旋转擦拭尿道口、龟头及冠状沟。

9. 每个棉球限用一次。消毒完毕脱下手套，放入弯盘移至床尾。

10. 在病人两腿之间以无菌技术展开导尿包，戴无菌手套。

11. 铺洞巾于病人会阴部，暴露尿道口。

12. 打开所有用物包装袋：

（1）打开集尿袋，取出并捋直引流管，确认集尿袋完好。

（2）打开其他包装袋，取出用物。

（3）连接载水注射器和导尿管，检查气囊有无漏气。

（4）连接导尿管和引流袋。

（5）如为女性病人导尿，需润滑导尿管前端 2.5～5 cm，男病人为 15～17.5 cm。

13. 再次消毒尿道口。

（1）女性病人：

操作者一手分开并固定小阴唇，充分暴露尿道口。另一手持镊子夹取消毒液棉球，（由内向外，从上到下）依次消毒尿道口、两侧小阴唇，最后再次消毒尿道口。每个棉球限用一次。

（2）男性病人：

同初步消毒法，一手握住阴茎，另一手持镊子夹取消毒液棉球，以尿道口为中心旋转擦拭尿

meatus down to the glans penis and the coronal sulcus in a circular motion. Use a new cotton ball each time and repeat it three times. Avoid returning the foreskin over the cleansed meatus or letting go of the penis.

14. Place the used forceps and cotton balls in the kidney dish and move the dish away from the perineum, but keep the dish within the aseptic area.

15. Move the collection container with the catheter to the perineum.

16. Insert the catheter：

（1）Use plain tissue forceps to hold the catheter 5-7 cm from the tip. Ask the patient to take a deep breath and insert the catheter as the patient exhales.

（2）When urine drains out, advance the catheter 7-10 cm further. **Rationale**：*This is to guarantee the balloon is fully in the bladder and will not easily fall out*. For male patients, hold the penis at 60° towards the patient's abdomen before insertion. **Rationale**：*Lifting the penis in this manner helps straighten the urethra*.

（3）If the catheter accidentally contacts the labia or slips into the vagina, it is considered contaminated and a new sterile catheter must be used. In order to avoid mistaking again, the contaminated catheter can be left in the vagina until the new catheter is inserted.

17. Move your non-dominant hand down to hold the catheter between the last two fingers and the balloon port between the first two fingers. In the meanwhile, attach the syringe and inflate the balloon with the designated volume of sterile water with your dominant hand.

18. Pull gently on the catheter until resistance is felt to ensure the balloon has inflated and placed in the trigone of the bladder.

19. Collect a midstream urine specimen if needed：

（1）Allow forepart urine to flow into the urine bag, and close the clamp.

（2）Fold the urine drainage port with the non-

道口、龟头及冠状沟,重复消毒三次,每个棉球限用一次。勿使包皮回缩及阴茎滑落。

14.用过的镊子和棉球放入弯盘内,移开,但仍在无菌区内。

15.将盛有导尿管的盘子移近会阴处。

16.插导尿管:

(1)用平镊夹持距离导尿管头端5～7 cm处,嘱病人深呼吸,于病人呼气时插入导尿管。

(2)见尿液流出后再插入7～10 cm。**依据**:确保导尿管和气囊在膀胱内,不易滑出。男性病人插管前提起阴茎与腹壁成60°角。**依据**:使尿道变直。

(3)如导尿管不慎触及阴唇或误入阴道,应视为污染,须更换导尿管重新插入。为避免再次误插,误入阴道的导尿管暂时保留在内,待新的导尿管插入尿道后再拔出误入阴道的导尿管。

17.松开固定小阴唇的手,下移,用其最后两手指夹住固定导尿管,拇指和食指握住导尿管气囊口,另一手取载水注射器向气囊内注入指定容量的灭菌用水使气囊膨胀。

18.轻拉导尿管直到有阻力感,即证实导尿管气囊已膨胀并在膀胱三角内。

19.需要时留取中段尿:

(1)待前段尿液引流至集尿袋后夹闭引流管。

(2)用非惯用手折起导尿管

dominant hand and disconnect it from the urine bag.

(3) Allow 5～10 mL urine to flow into the bottle. Avoid the catheter orifice touching the bottle.

(4) Connect the tubing and the catheter again after collecting.

20. For an intermittent catheter，deflate the balloon and remove the catheter after urine flow stops.

21. For an indwelling catheter，remove the fenestrated drape and hang the bag below the level of the bladder. Open the clamp. Keep the tubing above the top of the bag (see Figure 14-4).

引流接口,分离导尿管和集尿袋。

(3)收集 5～10 mL 尿标本,导尿管连接口勿触及标本瓶口。

(4)尿标本收集完毕,连接导尿管和引流管。

20. 如为一次性导尿,导尿完毕即可抽空气囊,拔除导尿管。

21. 如是留置导尿,撤去孔巾,挂引流袋于床沿,低于膀胱水平。引流管应始终高于引流袋上缘(见图 14-4)。

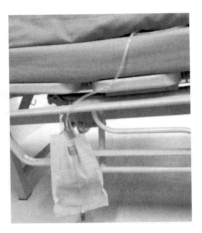

Figure 14-4　Correct position for the urine drainage bag and the tubing

图 14-4　集尿袋和引流管的悬挂

22. Wipe any remaining antiseptic from the patient's perineal area. Remove the protective pad, and move away all used supplies.

23. Remove and discard the gloves.

24. Remove the bath towel.

25. Assist the patient in putting on the trousers and place the patient in a comfortable position. Replace the foreskin if it was retracted earlier.

26. Perform hand hygiene.

27. Label the catheter，indicating the name of the catheter and the date of insertion.

28. Perform hand hygiene again.

29. Instruct the patient to position and move with the catheter keeping in place.

22. 擦干外阴部残留的消毒液。撤出护理垫及其用物。

23. 脱下手套,弃置。

24. 撤去浴巾。

25. 协助病人穿好裤子,躺卧舒适。男性病人将其包皮回复。

26. 洗手。

27. 在导尿管上贴标签,注明导管名称、插管日期。

28. 再次洗手。

29. 指导病人翻身或移动体位时防止导尿管脱出。

30. Discard all used supplies appropriately.

31. Record the catheterization results.

**EVALUATION**

• Teach the patient how to care for the indwelling catheter，tell him/her to drink more water，and provide other related interventions.

30. 合理处置用物。

31. 记录导尿结果。

**评价**

• 指导病人留置导尿管的护理方法、多饮水及其他相关的护理措施。

# Words and Expressions

catheterization *n.* 导管插入

collapse *n.* 病倒；*vt.*（尤指病重而）倒下，晕倒

coronal *adj.* 冠状的；*n.* 冠状物

coronal sulcus 冠状沟

designated *adj.* 指定的，认定的

distend *vi.* 肿胀，膨胀；*vt.*（使）膨胀，肿胀

distension *n.* 膨胀，肿胀

fenestrated *adj.* 有孔的，有窗的

fenestrated drape 洞巾，有孔巾

Foley catheter 福莱导尿管（气囊导尿管）

foreskin *n.* 包皮

frail *adj.* 瘦弱的，易损的

glans *n.* 龟头，阴茎头，阴蒂头

glans penis 龟头

hematuria *n.* 血尿

incision *n.* 割口，（尤指手术的）切口

indwelling/retention catheterization 留置导尿

irrigation *n.* 冲洗（伤口或身体部位）

labia *n.* 阴唇

labia majora 大阴唇

meatus *n.* ［解剖］口，道

midstream *n.* 中流，河流中心

mons pubis *n.* 阴阜

pelvic *adj.* 骨盆的

penis *n.* 阴茎

perineal *adj.* ［解剖］会阴的

perineum *n.* ［解剖］会阴

prefill *vt.* 预先充满，预装填

scrotum *n.* 阴囊

sulcus *n.* 沟，槽，裂缝

trigone *n.* 膀胱三角区，三角区

urethra *n.* 尿道

urethral *adj.* 尿道的

urinary tract infection（UTI）尿路感染

urine *n.* 尿，小便

vagina *n.* 阴道

# SKILL 15 Withdrawing Medication from Ampules

An ampule is usually made of clear glass and has a distinctive shape with a constricted neck. An ampule often has a colored dot above the neck which identifies the location of small cut in the glass to help break/open the ampule. Nurses should prevent hand injuries from the broken glass when breaking the ampule neck.

二维码 15-1

## PURPOSE

- To make preparations for an injection.

## PLANNING

- Aseptic techniques should be followed at all times to prevent cross-contamination.

### Equipment

1. Patient's MAR or computer printout
2. Ampule medication (see Figure 15-1)
3. File
4. Sterile syringe and needle of the proper size (see Figures 15-2，15-3)
5. Antiseptic swabs
6. Sterile gauze squares or cotton balls
7. Alcohol-based hand rub
8. Sharp container

# 技能操作 15 自安瓿抽吸药液法

安瓿一般由透明玻璃制成，其上有一缩窄颈部。安瓿颈上方有一颜色标记点，指示此处颈部已划割、可掰断安瓿。护士在掰安瓿时应防止手被玻璃割伤。

二维码 15-2

## 目的

- 为注射做准备。

## 计划

- 始终遵守无菌操作原则，防止交叉感染。

### 用物准备

1. 病人给药单或电脑打印单
2. 安瓿药液（见图 15-1）
3. 砂轮
4. 型号合适的无菌注射器和针头（见图 15-2、图 15-3）
5. 消毒液棉签
6. 无菌纱布块或棉球
7. 速干手消毒剂
8. 利器盒

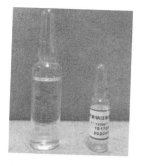

Figure 15-1  Ampules
图 15-1  安瓿

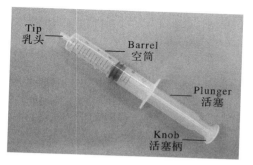

Figure 15-2  The four parts of a syringe
图 15-2  注射器结构

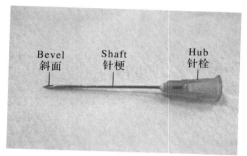

Figure 15-3  The three parts of a needle
图 15-3  针头结构

## IMPLEMENTATION

### Preparation

1. Perform hand hygiene and put on a mask.
2. Check the sterility of the equipment.
3. Check the MAR.
4. Check the medication:

(1) Carefully read the label on the ampule against the MAR three times to make sure that you have the correct medication:

1) when the ampule is taken out from the medication store;

2) before withdrawing the medication;

3) after withdrawing the medication.

(2) Check the expiration date and quality of the medication.

(3) Ask another staff to check the medication against the MAR.

## 实施

### 准备

1. 洗手,戴口罩。
2. 确定用物有效。
3. 核对给药单。
4. 核对药液:

(1) 根据给药单信息核对药物标签,仔细进行三查以确保药物正确:

1) 药物从药柜取出时;

2) 抽药前;

3) 抽药后。

(2) 检查药液有效期和质量。

(3) 二人核对无误。

5. Organize the equipment.

## Procedure

1. Prepare the ampule for medication withdrawal：

(1) Flick the top of the ampule several times with a fingernail (see Figure 15-4). **Rationale**：*This will bring all medication down to the ampule body.*

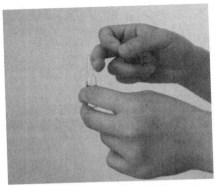

Figure 15-4　　Flicking the ampule head/top to bring the medication down

图 15-4　轻弹安瓿头使药液流至安瓿体

(2) Partially file the neck of the ampule if needed，and wipe the neck with an antiseptic swab.

(3) Place a piece of sterile gauze or a cotton ball around the ampule head and break it by bending the neck to the opposite side of the colored mark (see Figure 15-5). **Rationale**：*The sterile gauze protects the fingers from the broken glass，and provents any glass fragment from spraying away.*

(4) Dispose of the top of the ampule in the sharp container.

2. Withdraw the medication：

(1) Ensure the sterility of the syringe before opening the package.

(2) Attach the needle tightly to the syringe，and remove the needle cap.

(3) Insert the needle into the ampule with the bevel downward，and place it under the surface of the medication. Slightly tilt the ampule and withdraw the

5. 备齐用物。

## 操作步骤

1. 安瓿准备：

(1) 用一手指甲轻弹安瓿头(见图 15-4)。**依据**：使安瓿头部的药液流至安瓿体部。

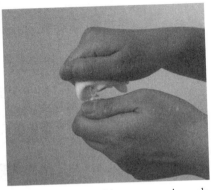

Figure 15-5　Breaking an ampule neck

图 15-5　掰安瓿法

(2) 必要时用砂轮在安瓿颈部划一锯痕，用消毒液棉签擦拭安瓿颈。

(3) 用一无菌纱布块或棉球包绕安瓿头，向标识点对侧掰断安瓿(见图 15-5)。**依据**：无菌纱布块可防止手指划割及玻璃碎片弹出。

(4) 将安瓿头置入利器盒。

2. 抽吸药液：

(1) 确定注射器的无菌性后打开包装。

(2) 紧密连接注射器与针头，取下护针帽。

(3) 针头斜面向下，伸入安瓿内的液面下，将安瓿稍倾斜，手持活塞柄，抽动活塞，抽吸药液

medication by pulling the plunger of the syringe, touching only its knob (see Figure 15-6, 15-7).

（见图 15-6、图 15-7）。

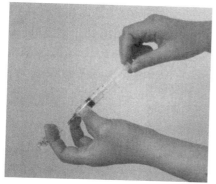

Figure 15-6 Withdrawing the medication from a small ampoule

图 15-6 自小安瓿抽吸药液法

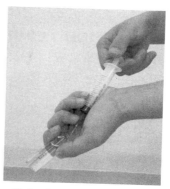

Figure 15-7 Withdrawing the medication from a big ampoule

图 15-7 自大安瓿抽吸药液法

(4) After withdrawal, invert the syringe, gently pull the plunger to bring the medication in the needle shaft down to the syringe, and expel the air while remaining the needle shaft within the empty ampule.

（4）抽吸完毕，倒转注射器，轻拉活塞，使针梗内药液流入注射器，轻推活塞，排出空气（针头在空安瓿内）。

## EVALUATION

• Check if the dosage is accurate and the medication, syringe and needle are not contaminated.

## 评价

• 抽吸剂量准确，药液、注射器和针头未污染。

## Words and Expressions

ampule/ampoule *n.* 安瓿

bevel *n.* 斜边，斜面

constricted *adj.* 紧缩的，缩窄的，限制的

distinctive *adj.* 有特色的，特别的

dosage *n.* （通常指药的）剂量

expel *vt.* 排出，喷出

file *n.* 锉刀，文件夹；*vt.* 锉去，锉薄

flick *vt.* （尤指用手指或手快速地）轻弹，轻击

knob 活塞柄

medication administration record （MAR）给药单

shaft *n.* 轴，杆

sharp container 利器盒

withdrawal *n.* 抽吸

# SKILL 16  Withdrawing Medication from Vials

A drug in the vial can be either liquid or powder. A powdered medication must be dissolved in liquid（solvents）before it can be injected. Commonly used diluents are sterile water and sterile normal saline. Some drugs have their specific solvents. Dissolved drugs have to be used within a certain period of time，and thus the date and time of dissolution should be written on the label of the vial. Nurses need to observe the expiration date.

二维码 16-1

## PURPOSE

- To make preparations for an injection.

## PLANNING

### Equipment

1. Patient's MAR or computer printout
2. Vial of sterile medication（see Figure 16-1）
3. Antiseptic swabs
4. Sterile syringe and needle of the proper size
5. Medication solvents if the drug is in powdered form（e. g.，sterile water，normal saline，specific solvents）
6. Vial opener
7. Alcohol-based hand rub
8. Sharp container

# 技能操作 16  自密封瓶抽吸药液法

密封瓶装药物可呈液体状或粉状。粉状药物需经溶媒溶解后方能注射。常用的溶媒有灭菌注射用水和无菌生理盐水，而某些药物有其特定溶媒。药物溶解后应在规定时间内使用，护士须在药物标签上注明溶解时间，并注意失效时间。

二维码 16-2

## 目的

- 为注射做准备。

## 计划

### 用物准备

1.病人给药单或电脑打印单
2.无菌密封瓶药物（见图 16-1）
3.消毒液棉签
4.型号合适的无菌注射器和针头
5.如为粉状药物，准备药物溶媒（如灭菌注射用水、生理盐水、专用溶媒）
6.启瓶器
7.速干手消毒剂
8.利器盒

# IMPLEMENTATION

## Preparation

- Follow the preparation procedure as described in Skill 15.

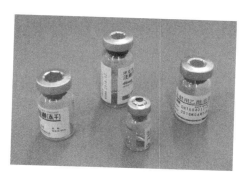

Figure 16-1　Vials
图 16-1　密封瓶

## Procedure

1. Prepare the vial medication for withdrawal：

(1) Remove the metal (with the vial opener) or plastic cap of the vial. Clean the rubber stopper with an antiseptic swab by rubbing in a circular motion.

(2) Firmly attach the needle to the syringe. Remove the needle cap.

(3) If the medication is in powdered form，withdraw sterile water or normal saline (or its specific solvent) into the syringe. Insert the needle into the center of the rubber stopper and inject the liquid，and maintain the sterility of the needle. Shake well to dissolve the medication.

(4) Check the quality of the medication.

2. Withdraw the medication：

(1) Draw into the syringe the amount of air equal to the volume of the medication to be withdrawn.

(2) Insert the needle into the center of the rubber stopper.

(3) Hold the vial in the same way as holding a big ampule. Inject the air into the vial (see Figure 16-2). **Rationale**：*The air will allow the medication*

# 实施

## 准备

- 同技能操作 15 的"准备"。

## 操作步骤

1. 准备密封瓶药物：

(1)除去密封瓶上的金属(用启瓶器)或塑料瓶盖,用消毒液棉签以螺旋形动作擦拭橡胶塞。

(2)紧密连接注射器与针头,取下护针帽。

(3)如为粉状药物,注射器内抽灭菌注射用水或生理盐水(或专用溶媒),针头由橡胶塞中心刺入瓶内并注入药物溶媒,保持针头无菌。摇匀溶解药物。

(4)检查药液质量。

2.抽吸药液：

(1)注射器内抽取与所需药液等量的空气。

(2)将针头由橡胶塞中心刺入瓶内。

(3)似握大安瓿法握住密封瓶,注入空气(见图 16-2)。**依据**:注入空气使瓶内形成正压,易

to be drawn out easily because negative pressure will *not be created inside the vial.*

（4）Invert the vial. Ensure the needle tip is below the fluid level, and gradually withdraw the medication. **Rationale**：*Keeping the tip of the needle below the fliud level prevents air from being drawn into the syringe.*

（5）Hold the syringe and vial at eye level to withdraw the correct volume of the medication into the syringe (see Figure 16-3). Inject air at the top of the syringe back into the vial.

于抽取药液。

（4）倒转密封瓶使针头在液面下，缓慢抽吸药液。**依据**：保持针头在液面下，以防抽到空气。

（5）持注射器和密封瓶于视线水平，抽吸药液至所需量（见图 16-3）。将注射器上端空气注回密封瓶内。

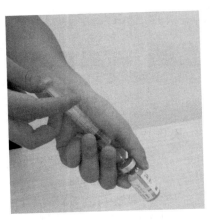

Figure 16-2　Injecting air into a vial

图 16-2　向密封瓶内注入空气

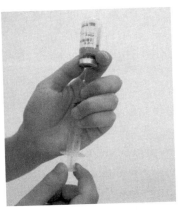

Figure 16-3　Withdrawing the medication from a vial

图 16-3　自密封瓶抽吸药液

（6）When the correct volume of medication is obtained, remove the needle from the vial. Recap the needle using the scoop method to prevent needle-stick injuries, while the needle should be kept sterile.

（7）If necessary, tap the syringe barrel to dislodge any air bubble present in the syringe. **Rationale**：*The tapping motion will cause the air bubbles to rise to the top of the syringe where they can be ejected out of the syringe.*

（8）If full dose of medication is needed, insert the whole shaft of the needle back into the vial to maintain its sterility before injection.

## EVALUATION

- Check if the dosage is accurate and the medication, syringe and needle are not contaminated.

（6）抽取所需剂量的药液后拔出针头，单手回套针头，防止针刺伤并保持针头无菌。

（7）必要时用手指拍注射器空筒气泡所在部位使其脱落。**依据**：使气泡上浮至乳头部位，以利于排气。

（8）如需全剂药液，注射前将针梗全部刺入密封瓶内以保持针头无菌。

## 评价

- 药液剂量抽吸准确，药液、注射器和针头无污染。

# Words and Expressions

dislodge *v.* 逐出,驱逐出,取出,移动

dissolution *n.* 分解,溶解

dissolve *vt.* 使溶解

dose *n.* 药的一剂,一服

needle-stick 针刺

solvent *n.* 溶媒,溶剂

tap *v.* 轻打

vial *n.* 玻璃小瓶,小药瓶

# SKILL 17　Administering an Intradermal Injection for Skin Tests

# 技能操作 17 皮内注射药物 过敏试验法

Certain medications tend to cause anaphylactic reaction in people with allergies. Correct diagnoses that based on valid allergy tests can help confirm or rule out allergies and avoid the adverse consequences.

某些药物会使过敏体质者产生过敏反应。根据有效的过敏试验进行正确的判断，有助于确定病人对该药物是否过敏，以避免不良后果的产生。

二维码 17-1

二维码 17-2

## PURPOSE

- To provide allergy tests for the medication that the patient needs.

## ASSESSMENT

1. Assess the patient's condition, consciousness and ability to cooperate.

2. Assess the patient's knowledge of and allergies to medication(s).

3. Assess skin condition of the selected site.

## PLANNING

### Equipment

1. Patient's MAR or computer printout
2. Vial or ampule of the correct medication
3. File or vial opener
4. Sterile 1-mL syringe, needle size $4^{1/2}$
5. 75% alcohol swabs
6. Sterile gauze squares or cotton balls
7. Clean gloves

## 目的

- 对所需药物做皮肤过敏试验。

## 评估

1. 病人的病情、意识状态及配合程度。

2. 病人的药物知识及药物过敏史。

3. 注射部位皮肤状况。

## 计划

### 用物准备

1. 病人给药单或电脑打印单
2. 安瓿或密封瓶药液
3. 砂轮或密封瓶启瓶器
4. 无菌 1 mL 注射器，$4^{1/2}$ 针头
5. 75% 酒精棉签
6. 无菌纱布块或棉球
7. 清洁手套

8. 0.1% epinephrine

9. Alcohol-based hand rub

10. Sharp container

## IMPLEMENTATION

### Preparation

1. Follow the preparation procedure as described in Skill 15.

2. Withdraw the medication from the ampule or vial as described in Skill 15 or Skill 16.

### Procedure

1. Carry the equipment to the bedside.

2. Before performing the procedure，introduce yourself and verify the patient's identity.

3. Explain to the patient that the injection will produce a small bleb. **Rationale**：*Information can facilitate acceptance and compliance of the patient to the therapy.*

4. Select and clean the injection site：

（1）Select the lower inner forearm as the injection site.

（2）Avoid using sites which are painful，inflamed or swollen，and which have other lesions.

（3）Put on gloves. **Rationale**：*This prevents the spread of pathogenic microorganisms and reduces the likelihood of contacting the patient's blood.*

5. Cleanse the skin of the site using an alcohol swab，starting at the center and moving outward in a circular manner with the diameter of about 5 cm. Allow the area to dry thoroughly.

6. Check the medication，and verify the patient's identity.

7. Prepare the syringe for injection. Remove the needle cap.

8. Expel air bubbles from the syringe. Small bubbles that adhere to the plunger are of no consequence. **Rationale**：*A small amount of air will not harm the tissues.*

9. Hold the syringe in your dominant hand between

8. 0.1% 盐酸肾上腺素针

9. 速干手消毒剂

10. 利器盒

## 实施

### 准备

1. 同技能操作 15 的"准备"。

2. 按技能操作 15 或技能操作 16 抽吸所需药液。

### 操作步骤

1. 携用物至床旁。

2. 操作前自我介绍,确认病人。

3. 向病人解释注射后会有一皮丘生成。**依据:**向病人提供信息可提高其对治疗的接受度和依从性。

4. 选择并消毒注射部位:

（1）选择前臂掌侧下段作为注射部位。

（2）避免在疼痛、炎症、肿胀或有其他病变的部位注射。

（3）戴清洁手套。**依据:**防止病原微生物传播及降低接触病人血液的概率。

5. 用酒精棉签以注射点为中心,向外旋转涂擦消毒皮肤,直径约 5 cm,待干。

6. 检查药物,确认病人。

7. 准备好注射器,取下护针帽。

8. 排尽注射器内空气。小气泡可忽略。**依据:**小气泡对组织无损害。

9. 用惯用手的手指握住注

your fingers. Hold the needle almost parallel to the skin surface, with the bevel of the needle up. **Rationale**: *The possibility of the medication entering the subcutaneous tissue increases when using an angle greater than 15°.*

10. Inject the fluid:

(1) With the non-dominant hand, pull the skin taut over the injection site (see Figures 17-1, 17-2). **Rationale**: *Taut skin allows for easier entry of the needle and brings less discomfort to the patient.*

射器,针头斜面向上,与皮肤几乎平行。**依据**:进针角度＞15°可使药液注入皮下组织。

10. 注射药液:

(1) 用非惯用手绷紧注射部位皮肤(见图17-1、图17-2)。**依据**:绷紧皮肤易于进针并可减轻病人不适。

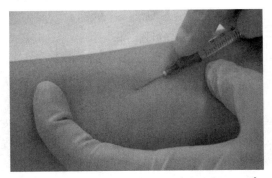

Figure 17-1　The needle enters the skin at 5° (pulling the skin taut with two fingers)

图17-1　针头斜面与皮肤成5°角刺入皮内(两手指绷皮肤)

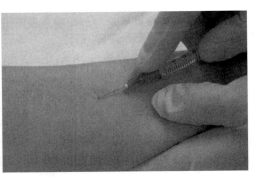

Figure 17-2　The needle enters the skin at 5° (pulling the skin taut with one finger)

图17-2　针头斜面与皮肤成5°角刺入皮内(用拇指绷皮肤)

(2) Place the needle against the skin at 5°, with the bevel up, and insert the needle through the epidermis into dermis until the bevel is completely in.

(3) Place the syringe flat against the skin. Stabilize the needle hub and tip of the syringe with the non-dominant thumb. Slowly inject 0.1 mL of the medication until a small bleb appears (see Figure 17-3). **Rationale**: *This verifies that the medication entered the dermis.*

(4) Quickly withdraw the needle at the same angle.

(5) Do not massage the area. **Rationale**: *Massage can disperse the medication into the tissue or make it flow out of the injection site.*

(6) Dispose of the needle into the sharp container. **Rationale**: *Do not recap the needle so as to prevent needle-stick injuries.*

(2) 针头斜面与皮肤成5°角自表皮刺入,直至针尖斜面完全进入皮内。

(3) 放平注射器,用绷紧皮肤的手拇指固定注射器乳头和针栓。缓慢注入0.1 mL药液,使局部隆起形成一皮丘(见图17-3)。**依据**:皮丘生成表明药液已注入皮内。

(4) 注射完毕,按注射时的角度快速拔出针头。

(5) 勿按压针眼。**依据**:按压会使药液渗入皮下组织或自针眼流出。

(6) 将针头置入利器盒。**依据**:勿回套护针帽,避免针刺伤。

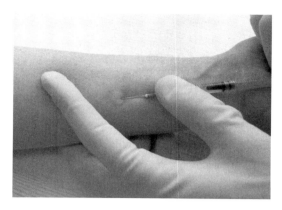

Figure 17-3　The medication forms a bleb under the epidermis

图 17-3　药液注入皮内形成皮丘

（7）Remove and discard the gloves.

（8）Mark the injection site with a pen and write down the due time（after 20 min）.

11. Confirm the patient and check the medication again.

12. Perform hand hygiene.

13. Provide appropriate instructions.

14. Document all relevant information: the injection time, drug name, dosage, route, etc.

## EVALUATION

● Evaluate the patient's reaction to the medication. Some medications used in testing may cause allergic reaction. Emergency drugs（e. g. , epinephrine）must be around.

（7）脱下手套、弃置。

（8）用笔标记皮丘部位,注明到点时间（20 分钟后）。

11. 再次确认病人,核对药物。

12. 洗手。

13. 交代注意事项。

14. 记录注射时间、药名、剂量、给药途经等。

## 评价

● 评价病人对药物的反应。某些皮试液会引起过敏,皮试前必须备好急救药品（如肾上腺素针）。

# Words and Expressions

anaphylactic *adj.* 过敏反应的

bleb *n.* 水泡,气泡

consequence *n.* 结果,后果

dermis *n.* 真皮

disperse *vt.* 分散,传播,散开

epidermis *n.* 表皮

epinephrine *n.* 肾上腺素

hub *n.* 针栓,冲头

inflamed *adj.* 发炎的,红肿的

inner forearm 前臂掌侧

intradermal/intradermic *adj.* 真皮内的,皮肤内的

intradermal injection（ID）皮内注射

lesion *n.* 损害,损伤

rule out 把……排除在外

stabilize *vt.*（使）稳固,稳定

swollen *adj.* 肿胀的,浮肿的

taut *adj.* 拉紧的,绷紧的

# SKILL 18　Administering an Intramuscular Injection

Injections into the muscle are absorbed more quickly and in a larger volume than subcutaneous injections because of the greater blood supply to the muscle tissue while causing less discomfort. A major consideration in the administration of intramuslular(IM) injections is the selection of a safe site located away from large blood vessels，large nerves and bones. The ventrogluteal site is the safest site for IM injections in patients older than 7 months. This is because it contains no large nerves or large blood vessels，but the use of this site for IM injections in clinical practice is infrequent.

二维码 18-1

## PURPOSE

- To provide medication that the patient needs.

## ASSESSMENT

1. Assess the patient's condition，consciousness，ability or willingness to cooperate.

2. Assess the patient's knowledge of medication and allergy history.

3. Check skin and tissue integrity of the selected site.

4. Assess the patient's age and weight to determine injection site and needle size.

## PLANNING

### Equipment

1. Patient's MAR or computer printout

# 技能操作 18 肌内注射法

因肌肉组织血液供应较丰富,药液经肌内注射比皮下注射吸收更迅速,吸收量更大,而不适感较轻。肌内注射部位应远离大血管、大神经和骨骼。7 个月以上的病人以臀中肌、臀小肌部位注射最安全,因该部位不含大神经和大血管。但是临床实践中较少在该部位进行肌内注射。

二维码 18-2

## 目的

- 供给病人药物。

## 评估

1. 病人的病情、意识状态、配合程度或意愿。

2. 病人的药物知识及药物过敏史。

3. 注射部位皮肤及肌肉组织的完整性。

4. 病人年龄及体重,以确定注射部位和针头型号。

## 计划

### 用物准备

1. 病人给药单或电脑打印单

2. Vial or ampule medication

3. Sterile syringe and needle of the proper size

4. File or vial opener

5. 0.5% iodophors/Betadine swabs

6. Sterile swabs

7. Sterile gauze squares or cotton balls

8. Clean gloves

9. Alcohol-based hand rub

10. Sharp container

## IMPLEMENTATION

### Preparation

1. Follow the preparation procedure as described in Skill 15.

2. Withdraw the medication from the ampule or vial as described see Skill 15 or Skill 16.

### Procedure

1. Carry the equipment to the bedside.

2. Before performing the procedure, introduce yourself and verify the patient's identity.

3. Explain to the patient the purpose for and the effects of the medication.

4. Protect the patient's privacy.

5. Assist the patient to take a supine, lateral, prone or sitting position, depending on the chosen site. Get assistance when the patient is unable to cooperate.

6. Select, locate and clean the site:

(1) Select a site free of skin lesions, pain, swelling, hardness or inflammation and having not been used frequently.

(2) Dorsogluteal muscle: The patient needs to take a side-lying position with the upper leg straight and lower leg flexed (or a prone position with the toes pointed towards each other and heels separated). **Rationale**: *Appropriate positioning promotes relaxation of the target muscle.*

(3) Ventrogluteal muscle: The patient lies on

2. 安瓿或密封瓶药液

3. 型号合适的无菌注射器和针头

4. 砂轮或密封瓶启瓶器

5. 0.5%碘伏棉签

6. 无菌棉签

7. 无菌纱布块或棉球

8. 清洁手套

9. 速干手消毒剂

10. 利器盒

## 实施

### 准备

1. 同技能操作 15 的"准备"。

2. 按技能操作 15 或技能操作 16 抽吸所需药液。

### 操作步骤

1. 携用物至床旁。

2. 操作前自我介绍并确认病人。

3. 向病人解释用药目的。

4. 保护病人隐私。

5. 根据所选注射部位,协助病人取仰、侧、俯卧或坐位。如病人不能合作,寻求助手。

6. 定位,消毒:

(1) 选择无皮肤损伤、疼痛、肿胀、硬结或炎症及注射次数较少的部位。

(2) 臀大肌注射:病人侧卧,大腿伸直,小腿弯曲(俯卧位:足尖相对,足跟分开)。**依据**:卧位适当可使肌肉松弛。

(3) 臀中肌、臀小肌注射:病

the back or on the side with the upper leg straight and the lower leg flexed.

（4）Vastus lateralis muscle：The patient lies on the back or take a sitting position.

（5）Deltoid muscle：The patient lies or sits with the arm flexed.

（6）Clean the site with a 0.5％ iodophors swab. Using a circular motion, start at the centre and gradually move outward with the diameter of about 5 cm.

（7）Hold a dry sterile swab between the third and fourth (or the fourth and fifth) fingers of your non-dominant hand in readiness for needle withdrawal, or position the swab on the patient's skin above the intended site. Allow skin to dry before injecting medication. **Rationale**：*This will help reduce the discomfort of the injection.*

7. Prepare the syringe for injection. Remove the needle cap. Ensure there is no air bubble in the syringe.

8. Verify the patient's identity, and check the medication.

9. Inject the medication：

（1）With the thumb and forefinger of the non-dominant hand, pull the skin taut over the injection site (see Figure 18-1).

（2）With the dominant hand, hold the syringe between the fingers, and quickly and smoothly inject 1/2-2/3 of the needle into the skin at 90° (see Figure 18-1). **Rationale**：*Using a quick motion lessens the patient's discomfort.* If necessary, use Z-track method.

人取仰卧或侧卧位，大腿伸直，小腿弯曲。

（4）股外侧肌注射：病人仰卧或坐位。

（5）三角肌注射：病人取仰卧位或坐位，手臂弯曲。

（6）用 0.5％ 碘伏棉签以注射点为中心向外旋转涂擦消毒皮肤，直径约 5 cm。

（7）非惯用手的第 3、4（或第 4、5）手指间夹一干棉签，或将棉签放于注射部位旁边，准备拔针时按压。注射部位待干。**依据**：可减轻病人不适。

7. 准备注射器，取下护针帽。确认注射器内无气泡。

8. 确认病人，核对药物。

9. 注射药液：

（1）用非惯用手的拇指和食指绷紧注射部位皮肤（见图 18-1）。

（2）惯用手持注射器，使针头与皮肤呈 90°角，平稳、迅速地刺入肌内（针梗的 1/2～2/3 长）（见图 18-1）。**依据**：快速进针可减轻疼痛。必要时利用"Z"形注射技术。

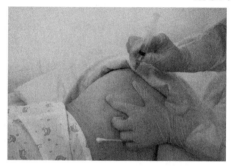

Figure 18-1　Administering an intramuscular injection into the dorsogluteal site

图 18-1　臀大肌注射法

(3) Using the same hand, hold the barrel of the syringe steady and aspirate by pulling back on the plunger handle using your non-dominant hand. Aspirate for 5-10 seconds. **Rationale**: *If the needle gets into a small blood vessel, it takes time for the blood to appear.*

(4) If blood appears in the syringe, withdraw the needle, discard the syringe, and prepare a new injection.

(5) If blood does not appear, inject the medication slowly and evenly (approximately 1 mL per 10 seconds) while holding the syringe steady. **Rationale**: *Injecting medication slowly promotes comfort and gives time for tissue to expand and begin absorption of the medication. Holding the syringe steady minimizes discomfort.*

(6) After injection, wait 10 seconds if using the ventrogluteal site. **Rationale**: *Waiting permits the medication to disperse into the muscle tissue, thus decreasing the patient's discomfort.*

10. Withdraw the needle:

(1) Withdraw the needle smoothly and quickly at the same angle of insertion. **Rationale**: *This minimizes tissue injury and patient's discomfort.*

(2) At the same time, apply gentle pressure with a dry swab. **Rationale**: *Use of an alcohol swab may cause pain or a burning sensation.*

(3) Do not massage the injection site. **Rationale**: *Massaging the site may cause the leakage of medication from the site and result in irritation.*

(4) If bleeding occurs, apply pressure with a dry sterile swab until it stops.

11. Dispose of the needle into the sharp container.

12. Remove and discard the gloves.

13. Verify the patient's identity and check the medication again.

14. Perform hand hygiene.

15. Document all relevant information: the time of administration, drug name, dosage, route, and the patient's reaction.

（3）用同一只手持稳注射器，另一只手回抽活塞，持续 5～10 秒以检查回血。**依据**：针头如进入小血管，回血需要一定时间。

（4）如有回血，拔出针头弃去，准备重新注射。

（5）如无回血，持稳注射器，缓慢、匀速注入药液（约 1mL/10 秒）。**依据**：缓慢注射可减轻病人不适，利于组织缓慢扩张以吸收药液。持稳注射器可减轻病人不适。

（6）臀大肌注射完毕，应停留 10 秒再拔针。**依据**：等待片刻可使药液渗入肌肉组织以减轻不适。

10. 拔针：

（1）按进针时的角度快速拔针。**依据**：相同角度拔针可减轻组织损伤，快速拔针可减轻病人不适。

（2）拔针时用干棉签按压注射点。**依据**：用酒精棉签按压可致病人疼痛或有烧灼感。

（3）勿揉。**依据**：按摩可致药液漏出刺激皮肤。

（4）如仍有出血，用无菌干棉签按压至血止。

11. 将针头置入利器盒。

12. 脱下手套、弃置。

13. 再次确认病人，核对药物。

14. 洗手。

15. 记录注射时间、药名、剂量、途经及病人反应。

## EVALUATION

1. Observe the expected effects of the medication.

2. Report to the doctor if any adverse reaction or side-effect occurs.

## 评价

1. 观察药物预期效果。

2. 如出现药物不良反应和副作用，报告医生。

## Words and Expressions

absorb *vt.* 吸收（液体、气体等）

Betadine *n.* 必妥碘

deltoid *n.* 三角肌；*adj.* 三角形的

deltoid muscle 三角肌

dorsogluteal *adj.* 臀外侧的

　　（前缀 dors-/dorso- 表示"背的"）

dorsogluteal muscle 臀大肌

intramuscular (IM) *adj.* 肌内的

iodophors *n.* 碘伏

lateralis *n.* 侧体

nerve *n.* 神经

subcutaneous/hypodermic *adj.* 皮下的

　　（前缀 sub- 表示"在……下方"）

subcutaneous injection 皮下注射

vastus *n.* 股肌

ventrogluteal *adj.* 腹侧的

　　（前缀 ventr-/ventro- 表示"腹，腹部"）

ventrogluteal muscle 臀中肌、臀小肌

# SKILL 19   Administering an Intravenous Injection

# 技能操作 19 静脉注射法

Intravenous injection is preferred when rapid effect of medication is required or when other routes are either possible or advisable. IV medications enter the patients' bloodstream directly through the vein, and in no way can it be withdrawn or terminate its action. Therefore, the nurse must take special care to avoid any error in the preparation of the drug and the calculation of the dosage, Therefore, the nurse must take special care to avoid any error in the preparation of the drug and the calculation of the dosage, observe the principles of medication administration.

当需要快速发挥药效、不能或不宜经其他途径给药时，可经静脉给药。静脉注射的药物直接通过静脉进入病人血流，不能撤回或终止药物的作用，因此，护士尤应注意避免用错药物用错剂量及遵守给药原则。

二维码 19-1

二维码 19-2

## PURPOSES

1. To achieve immediate effect of the medication.

2. To assist certain diagnostic tests by injecting medications.

## ASSESSMENT

1. Assess the patient's condition, consciousness and ability of cooperation.

2. Assess the patient's knowledge of the medication and history of drug allergies.

3. Check status of veins, skin condition of the venipuncture site and the mobility of the selected extremity.

4. Assess for allergy to latex (e. g. , tourniquet) or adhesive tape.

## 目的

1. 迅速发挥药效。

2. 注入药物以协助某些诊断性检查。

## 评估

1. 病人的病情、意识状态及配合程度。

2. 病人的药物知识及药物过敏史。

3. 穿刺部位静脉、皮肤状况及肢体活动度。

4. 是否对乳胶类（如压脉带）或胶布过敏。

## PLANNING

### Equipment

1. Patient's MAR or computer printout

2. Vial or ampoule of the correct medication

3. File or vial opener

4. Sterile syringe, needle and IV needle（see Figure 19-1) of the proper size

5. 0.5% iodophors swabs

6. Sterile gauze squares or cotton balls

7. Adhesive tape

8. Tourniquet (see Figure 19-2(a),(b))

9. Small pad

10. Disposable drape

11. Clean gloves

12. Alcohol-based hand rub

13. Sharp container

## 计划

### 用物准备

1. 病人给药单或电脑打印单

2. 所需安瓿或密封瓶药物

3. 砂轮或密封瓶启瓶器

4. 型号合适的无菌注射器、针头和静脉输液针（见图 19-1）

5. 0.5%碘伏棉签

6. 无菌纱布块或棉球

7. 胶布

8. 压脉带（见图 19-2(a),(b)）

9. 小垫枕

10. 一次性护理垫

11. 清洁手套

12. 速干手消毒剂

13. 利器盒

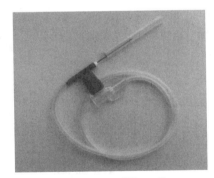

Figure 19-1　IV needle

图 19-1　静脉输液针

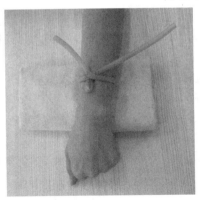
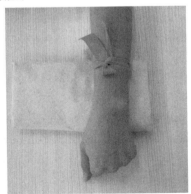

(a) 　　　　　　　　　　　　　(b)

Figure 19-2　Two types of tourniquets

图 19-2　两种止血带

## IMPLEMENTATION

### Preparation

1. Follow the preparation procedure as described in Skill 15.

2. Withdraw the medication from the ampule or vial as described in Skill 15 or Skill 16.

3. Connect the IV needle with the syringe，and expel the air in the needle tubing.

### Procedure

1. Carry the equipment to the bedside.

2. Prepare the patient：

（1）Before the procedure，verify the patient's identity by checking his/her identification band and asking his/her name. **Rationale**：*This ensures that the right patient receives the right medication.*

（2）Explain the purpose of administering the medication（how it will help），using language that the patient understands. **Rationale**：*Information can facilitate acceptance and compliance of the patient.*

3. Select the venipuncture site. Use the patient's non-dominant arm，unless contraindicated. Choose a vein which is relatively straight and distal to the wrist or elbow so that the tip of the needle will not be at a point of flexion. **Rationale**：*Joint flexion increases the risk of puncture of the vein by the needle.*

4. Wear clean gloves（this can be done before banding the tourniquet）. **Rationale**：*This reduces the transmission of microorganisms and reduces the likelihood of the nurses' hands contacting the patient's blood.*

5. Dilate the vein：

（1）Explain that the tourniquet will make the patient feel tight. Firmly band a tourniquet 6-8 cm above the venipuncture site. **Rationale**：*The tourniquet must be tight enough to obstruct venous flow but not so tight or it will occlude arterial flow.* The ends of the tourniquet face away from the injection site. **Rationale**：*This prevents the end of the tourniquet from touching the injection site*

## 实施

### 准备

1. 同技能操作 15 的"准备"。

2. 按技能操作 15 或技能操作 16 抽吸所需药液。

3. 连接注射器和静脉输液针,排气。

### 操作步骤

1. 携用物至床旁。

2. 病人准备：

（1）核对病人手腕带、询问病人姓名以确认病人。**依据**：确保病人正确,药物正确。

（2）使用通俗语言向病人解释给药目的、药物作用。**依据**：提供信息可提高病人对治疗的接受度和依从性。

3. 选择穿刺部位。如无禁忌,以注射非惯用手为宜,选择相对较直的静脉。注射部位勿靠近腕或肘关节以免针尖处于关节位置。**依据**：关节活动易使针尖戳破静脉。

4. 戴清洁手套。**依据**：减少微生物传播,降低护士双手接触病人血液的概率。

5. 充盈静脉：

（1）向病人说明扎压脉带有点紧。在穿刺点上方 6～8 cm 处扎压脉带。**依据**：压脉带松紧适宜,能使静脉充盈,又不阻断动脉血流。压脉带末端朝上。**依据**：防止压脉带末端触及已消毒的注射部位。

that has been disinfected.

（2）Avoid sharing the tourniquet to prevent cross-contamination.

（3）If the vein is not sufficiently dilated：

1）Massage the vein from distal to proximal in a centripetal motion. **Rationale**：*This action aids in filling the vein with blood*.

2）Ask the patient to clench and unclench the fist several times. **Rationale**：*Contracting the muscles compresses the distal veins, forcing blood to run along the veins and distend them*.

3）If the preceding steps fail to distend the vein, remove the tourniquet and wrap the extremity in a warm towel for 10-15 minutes. **Rationale**：*Heat dilates superficial blood vessels, causing them to fill*. Then repeat the steps to dilate the vein.

6. Clean the injection site in the same way as for IM injection. Before inserting the needle, allow the site to dry completely. Do not fan, blow, or wipe.

7. Prepare adhesive tape.

8. Clean the injection site again.

9. Verify the patient's identity, medication and route of administration.

10. Ensure there are no air bubbles in the tubing.

11. Insert the needle：

（1）Remove the protective cap of the needle.

（2）Hold the skin taut about 5 cm below the entry point by the non-dominant hand.

（3）Hold the needle wing (see Figure 19-3（a）,（b）,（c）) in the dominant hand, with the bevel of the needle up. Insert the needle into the vein at 15°-30°. When blood returns, decrease the angle until the needle is parallel to the vein and advance the needle for about 0.5-1 cm.

12. Release the tourniquet and ask the patient to unclench the fist.

13. Secure the needle with adhesive tape. Inject the medication slowly. After injection, quickly withdraw the needle. Meanwhile press the injection site

（2）一人一带，防止交叉感染。

（3）如静脉充盈不良：

1）向心方向由远到近揉搓静脉。**依据**：有助于静脉充盈。

2）嘱病人重复握拳、松拳几次。**依据**：握拳使肌肉收缩，压迫周围静脉，促进血液流动，从而使静脉充盈。

3）如上述方法仍不能使静脉充盈，则松开压脉带，用热毛巾敷于注射部位 10～15 分钟。**依据**：热可使浅表静脉扩张，使静脉充盈。再扎上压脉带。

6. 消毒方法同肌内注射。待干，勿煽、吹、擦。

7. 准备敷贴。

8. 再次消毒。

9. 核对病人、药物及给药途经。

10. 确认输液管内无气泡。

11. 进针：

（1）取下护针帽。

（2）操作者的非惯用手在穿刺部位下方约 5 cm 处绷紧皮肤。

（3）惯用手持针头（见图 19-3（a）,（b）,（c）），针尖斜面向上，与皮肤呈 15°～30°角刺入静脉，见回血后降低针头角度与静脉平行，再进针 0.5～1 cm。

12. 松开压脉带，嘱病人松拳。

13. 用胶布固定针头。缓慢注入药液，注射完毕，快速拔出针头，同时迅速下压敷贴至不出血

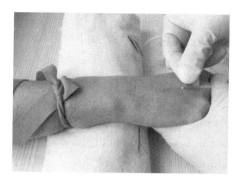

(a) Holding the needle wing with two fingers

(a) 两个手指持针翼

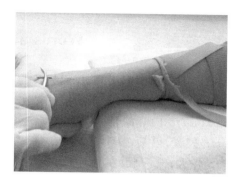

(b) Holding the needle wing with hemostats

(b) 血管钳持针翼

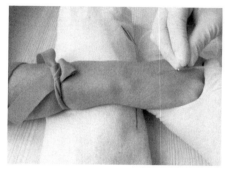

(c) Holding the needle wing with three fingers

(c) 三个手指持针翼

Figure 19-3　Three ways of holding the needle wing

图 19-3　持针翼的三种方法

immediately but gently until bleeding stops.

14. Verify the patient's identity，medication and route of administration again.

15. Dispose of the used equipment safely.

16. Remove and discard the gloves.

17. Perform hand hygiene.

18. Document relevant information.

## EVALUATION

1. Observe the patient closely for expected and adverse effects of the medication.

2. Report any significant change in the patient's condition to the doctor.

为止。

14. 再次核对病人、药物及给药途经。

15. 妥善处理用物。

16. 脱下手套、弃置。

17. 洗手。

18. 记录。

## 评价

1. 密切观察药物预期效果及不良反应。

2. 如病情出现较大变化,报告医生。

# Words and Expressions

aforementioned *adj.* 上述的，前面提及的

calculation *n.* 计算

centripetal *adj.* 向心的

clench *vt.* 捏紧，攥紧（拳头等）

dilate *vi.* 扩大；*vt.* （使）扩大，膨胀

error *n.* 错误，差错

flexion *n.* 弯曲，屈曲

terminate *vt.* （使）终止，结束

tourniquet *n.* 压脉带，止血带

venipuncture/venepuncture *n.* 静脉穿刺

# SKILL 20　Administering Peripheral Intravenous Infusion

# 技能操作 20
# 外周静脉输液法

Intravenous infusion is an efficient method of supplying fluids，electrolyte，and administering medications. Routes of intravenous infusion include deep line and peripheral line. A peripheral line is the most common type of IV therapy. The venipuncture site must be in the most distal portion of the arm because this allows for subsequent venipunctures to move upward. A deep line is used for infusions which need to be given rapidly and for solutions that are hypertonic or contain irritating medications. The venipuncture site varies with the patient's age，the duration and type of infusion，the type of medications used，and the condition of the veins.

静脉输液是一种迅速有效地补充水分、电解质及输入药物的方法，包括外周静脉和深静脉途经。外周静脉途经最常用，注射应从远心端静脉开始，逐渐向上选择和使用静脉。深静脉适用于需要快速输液或输入高浓度、刺激性强的药物。注射部位应根据病人年龄、输液所需时间、药物种类及静脉情况进行选择。

二维码 20-1

二维码 20-2

## PURPOSES

1. To supply fluids，balance electrolytes，and maintain the body's homeostasis.

2. To replenish circulating blood volume，improve microcirculation，and maintain blood pressure.

3. To provide substrates for metabolism.

4. To deliver medications to treat diseases.

## ASSESSMENT

1. Assess the patient's age，condition，consciousness and ability of cooperation.

2. Assess the patient's history of drug allergies.

3. Check status of veins，skin condition of the venipuncture site and the mobility of the extremity selected. Avoid sites which have been recently used.

## 目的

1. 补充水分及电解质，保持机体内环境稳定。

2. 增加循环血量，改善微循环，维持血压。

3. 提供机体新陈代谢所需基质。

4. 输入药物，治疗疾病。

## 评估

1. 病人年龄、病情、意识状态及配合程度。

2. 病人药物过敏史。

3. 穿刺部位静脉、皮肤状况及肢体活动度，避免在同一部位反复注射。

4. Assess allergy to latex (e. g. , tourniquet) or adhesive tape.

4. 是否对乳胶类（如压脉带）或胶布过敏。

## PLANNING

• Before IV infusion, consider what kind of medications and fluids will be given and how long the IV infusion will take to choose the needle size and the vein.

## 计划

• 操作前评估药物性质、溶液种类和输液所需时间，以选择合适的针头型号和输液部位。

### Equipment

1. Patient's MAR or computer printout

2. Correct sterile solution and medication
3. IV additive label
4. File or vial opener
5. Sterile syringe and needle of the appropriate size
6. Infusion set (see Figures 20-1, 20-2) with IV needle of the proper size (see Figure 19-1) or peripheral IV cannula (see Figure 20-3) (Choose the appropriate type and size based on the vein size and the purpose of IV. Always have spare IV needles or cannulas of both the same and different sizes. )
7. Adhesive tape
8. Transparent semipermeable membrane (TSM) dressing (if a peripheral IV cannula is used)
9. 0.5% iodophors swabs
10. Sterile gauze squares or cotton balls
11. Infusion observation card
12. Tourniquet
13. Small pad
14. Disposable drape
15. Clean bowl
16. Clean gloves
17. IV pole
18. Alcohol-based hand rub
19. Sharp container
20. Electronic infusion pump if required
21. Splint if required

### 用物准备

1. 病人输液医嘱单或电脑打印单

2. 所需无菌溶液及药物
3. 加药卡
4. 砂轮或密封瓶启瓶器
5. 型号合适的无菌注射器和针头
6. 输液器（见图 20-1、图 20-2）及型号合适的输液钢针（见图 19-1）或静脉留置针（见图 20-3）（根据静脉粗细及输液目的选择输液针头种类及型号，准备相同型号和不同型号的备用针头）
7. 胶布
8. 透明输液贴（使用静脉留置针时）
9. 0.5%碘伏棉签
10. 无菌纱布块或棉球
11. 输液观察卡
12. 压脉带
13. 小垫枕
14. 一次性护理垫
15. 清洁碗
16. 清洁手套
17. 输液架
18. 速干手消毒剂
19. 利器盒
20. 必要时备输液泵
21. 必要时备夹板

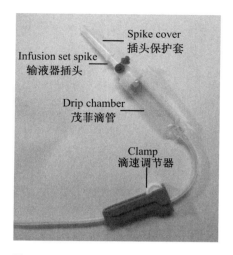

Figure 20-1  Parts of an IV infusion set
图 20-1  静脉输液器结构

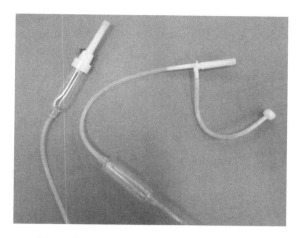

Figure 20-2  Two types of IV infusion sets
图 20-2  两种类型输液器

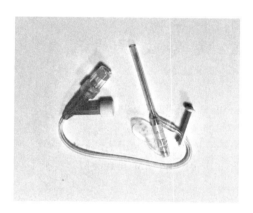

Figure 20-3  Peripheral IV cannula with dual port
图 20-3  周围静脉双腔留置计

## IMPLEMENTATION

### Preparation

1. Follow the preparation procedure as described in Skill 15.

2. Confirm compatibility of the drug and the solution being mixed.

3. Withdraw the medication from the ampule or vial as described in Skill 15 or Skill 16.

4. Check the solution as required.

5. Apply a medication label upside down on the

## 实施

### 准备

1.同技能操作 15 的"准备"。

2.确认无药物配伍禁忌。

3.按技能操作 15 或 16 抽吸所需药液。

4.按要求检查溶液质量。

5.将加药卡倒贴于溶液袋

solution bag(bottle). **Rationale**: *The label is applied upside down so it can be read easily when the bag(bottle) is hung up.* Do not cover the label of the solution.

6. Remove the lid of the solution bottle(bag) and clean the insertion site.

7. Add the medication:

(1) Inject the extracted medication into the bottle(bag), then withdraw air whose amount is equal to the volume of the medication injected.

(2) Mix the medication and solution by gently shaking the bag(bottle).

(3) Write down the time of adding medication, and sign your name on the label.

(4) Clean the insertion site of the solution bottle(bag) again.

8. Open and prepare the infusion set:

(1) Ensure the sterility of the infusion set before opening the package.

(2) Close the clamp.

(3) Remove the spike from the package (the tubing remains in the package).

(4) Remove the cap from the spike and insert the spike into the insertion site of the bottle(bag) completely.

9. Organize the equipment.

## Procedure

1. Carry the equipment to the bedside.

2. Prior to the procedure, introduce yourself and verify the patient's identity. Explain to the patient the purpose of administering the medication.

3. Ask the patient if he/she needs the toilet if the patient's condition permits. **Rationale**: *Moving the limb after the infusion was established could dislodge the needle(cannula).*

4. Perform hand hygiene, and put on a mask.

5. Check the solution and verify the patient's identity again.

（瓶）上。**依据**:输液袋(瓶)挂上后,加药卡倒贴易于查看。勿覆盖溶液瓶标签。

6.除去溶液袋(瓶)盖子,消毒注药口。

7.加药:

(1)将已抽好的药液注入溶液袋(瓶),抽出与注入药液等量的空气。

(2)轻轻摇动溶液袋(瓶)使药液混匀。

(3)在加药卡上注明加药时间并签名。

(4)再次消毒溶液袋(瓶)注药口。

8.准备输液器:

(1)确定输液器的无菌性后打开包装。

(2)夹闭调节器。

(3)取出输液器插头（皮管仍在包装袋内）。

(4)取下输液器插头的护套,将插头全部插入溶液袋(瓶)的注药口。

9.备齐用物。

## 操作步骤

1.携用物至床旁。

2.操作前自我介绍并确认病人,向病人解释输液目的。

3.询问病人是否需要上洗手间(病情允许者)。**依据**:肢体活动易使针头移位。

4.洗手,戴口罩。

5.再次检查溶液,确认病人。

6. To hang the solution bottle(bag) on the pole:

(1) Adjust the pole so that the bottle (bad) is suspended about 1 m above the patient's head. **Rationale**: *This height is needed to enable gravity to overcome venous pressure and facilitate flow of the solution into the vein.*

(2) Remove the tubing from the package and straighten it out.

7. Squeeze the drip chamber gently until it is half-filled with solution. **Rationale**: *The drip chamber is partially filled with solution to prevent air from moving down the tubing.*

8. Open the clamp and have the fluid run through the tubing until all air bubbles are removed (keep the needle cap in place). **Rationale**: *This will maintain the sterility of the needle.* If necessary, tap the tubing with your fingers where the bubbles are present to release them. **Rationale**: *Air bubbles less than 0.5 mL usually do not cause problems in peripheral lines.*

9. Reclamp the tubing and hang it on the IV pole.

10. Same as Steps 3-9 of Skill 19.

11. Ensure there are no air bubbles in the tubing.

12. Insert the needle. Same as Step 11 in Skill 19.

13. Release the tourniquet, unclamp the tubing and ask the patient to unclench his/her fist. Start the infusion.

14. Stabilize the needle:

(1) Secure the needle wing with tape, then loop the tubing and secure it with adhesive tape (see Figure 20-4(a),(b)).

(2) Apply a padded arm board to splint the joint if needed (see Figure 20-5).

(3) If an IV cannula is used, apply a TSM dressing over the site. Additional tape may be used to secure the IV cannula below the TSM. Label the tape with the date and the time of insertion, the cannula type, and your full name (see Figure 20-6).

6. 挂输液袋(瓶)于输液架上：

(1) 调节输液架,使溶液瓶(袋)高于病人头部约 1 m。**依据**:此高度使瓶(袋)内液压大于静脉压,使溶液滴入静脉。

(2)从输液器袋中取出皮管并捋直。

7. 挤压茂菲氏滴管使液面达滴管的 1/2 满。**依据**:滴管内有一定量的液体可防止空气进入下段输液管。

8. 打开调节器,使溶液流出直到管内气泡全部排出(勿去掉护针帽)。**依据**:保持针头无菌。必要时用手指轻弹输液管气泡所在部位协助排气。**依据**:<0.5 mL空气进入周围静脉对机体一般无损害。

9. 夹闭调节器,将输液管挂于输液架上。

10. 同技能操作 19 的步骤 3~9。

11. 确认输液管内无气泡。

12. 穿刺法同技能操作 19 的步骤 11。

13. 松开调节器和压脉带,嘱病人松拳(三松),开始输液。

14. 固定针头：

(1)用胶布固定针翼,再将针头软管环绕后固定 (见图 20-4 (a),(b))。

(2)必要时用夹板固定关节处(见图 20-5)。

(3)如使用静脉留置针,用透明输液贴固定针头,在透明输液贴下方再用胶布固定,上面标明注射日期、时间,签全名(见图 20-6)。

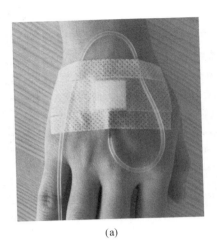 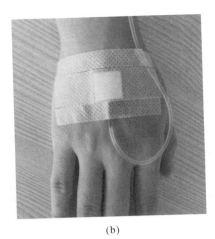

(a)　　　　　　　　　　　　　　(b)

Figure 20-4　Methods of securing the needle

图 20-4　针头固定法

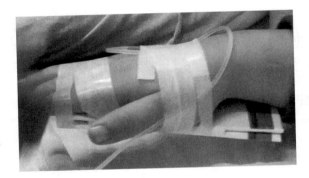 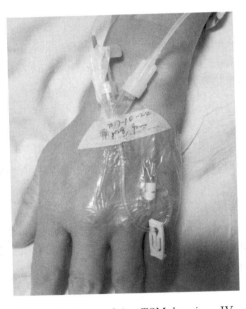

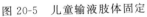

Figure 20-5　Immobilizing the extremity for cannulation of the hand in children

图 20-5　儿童输液肢体固定

Figure 20-6　Applying TSM dressing. IV site labeled with date, time, and staff's full name

图 20-6　用透明敷贴固定静脉留置针,注明注射日期、时间,签全名

15. Remove the tourniquet, and dispose of the used equipment safely.

16. Place the patient's arm properly.

17. Remove and discard the gloves.

15. 撤去压脉带,妥善处理用物。

16. 安置病人手臂。

17. 脱下手套、弃置。

18. Perform hand hygiene.

19. Slide the roller clamp along the tubing until it is just below the drip chamber to facilitate access (This can be done after finishing the procedure).

20. Adjust the infusion rate according to the patient's condition, age and medication properties (see Figure 20-7).

21. If an infusion pump is used, follow the manufacture's directions to place the tubing and set the infusion rate.

18. 洗手。

19. 将调节器拉至滴管下方便于操作。

20. 根据病人病情、年龄和药物性质调节输液滴速(见图 20-7)。

21. 如使用输液泵,应正确放置输液皮管及设置滴速。

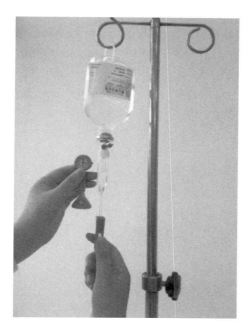

Figure 20-7　Adjusting the flow rate
图 20-7　调节滴速

22. Fill in the infusion observation card and hang it on the IV pole.

23. Notify the patient about the important matters related to the IV infusion.

24. Document all assessments and interventions in the patient's chart.

22. 填写输液观察卡,挂于输液架上。

23. 告知病人输液的注意事项。

24. 记录。

## EVALUATION

1. Regularly observe the patient for expected and adverse effects of the infusion.

## 评价

1. 定期观察药物预期效果及有无输液反应。

2. Regularly check the fluid level in the chamber and the infusion flow rate. Adjust the flow rate accordingly.

3. Check the skin condition at the IV site at least every 4 hours (redness, swelling, pain).

4. Report any significant change in the patients' condition to the doctor.

2. 定期检查滴管内液面及输液滴数，必要时调节。

3. 至少每 4 小时检查穿刺部位皮肤情况（有无红、肿、痛）。

4. 如病情出现较大变化，报告医生。

## Words and Expressions

cannulation *n.* 穿刺置管

compatibility *n.* 兼容性，相容性

compatible *adj.* 兼容的

electrolyte *n.* 电解质

homeostasis *n.* 体内稳态，内环境稳定

irritating *adj.* 刺激的

metabolism *n.* 新陈代谢

microcirculation *n.* 微循环

substrate *n.* 基质，底物

venous *adj.* 静脉的

# **References**
# 参考文献

［1］Berman A，Snyder S，Frandsen G. Kozier & Erb's fundamentals of nursing：concepts，process，and practice［M］. 10th ed. Hoboken：Pearson Education，Inc，2016.

［2］World Health Organization. WHO guidelines on hand hygiene in health care：first global patient safety challenge：clean care is safer care［M］. Geneva：World Health Organization，2009：152-156.

［3］冯志仙.护理技术操作程序与质量管理标准［M］.2 版.杭州:浙江大学出版社,2013.

［4］李小寒,尚少梅.基础护理学［M］.6 版.北京:人民卫生出版社,2017.

图书在版编目（CIP）数据

基础护理技能操作指导:汉英对照／练正梅主编.
—杭州:浙江大学出版社,2019.9(2025.1重印)
ISBN 978-7-308-19316-0

Ⅰ.①基… Ⅱ.①练… Ⅲ.①护理学－汉、英 Ⅳ.
①R47

中国版本图书馆 CIP 数据核字（2019）第 143412 号

**基础护理技能操作指导（中英双语版）**

练正梅　主编

| | |
|---|---|
| 丛书策划 | 阮海潮（1020497465@qq.com） |
| 责任编辑 | 阮海潮 |
| 责任校对 | 仲亚萍 |
| 封面设计 | 续设计 |
| 出版发行 | 浙江大学出版社 |
| | （杭州市天目山路 148 号　邮政编码 310007） |
| | （网址:http://www.zjupress.com） |
| 排　　版 | 浙江时代出版服务有限公司 |
| 印　　刷 | 杭州杭新印务有限公司 |
| 开　　本 | 787mm×1092mm　1/16 |
| 印　　张 | 9.25 |
| 字　　数 | 300 千 |
| 版 印 次 | 2019 年 9 月第 1 版　2025 年 1 月第 2 次印刷 |
| 书　　号 | ISBN 978-7-308-19316-0 |
| 定　　价 | 39.00 元 |